Epigenetics and Assisted Reproduction

An Introductory Guide

T0341197

Epigenetics and Assisted Reproduction
An Introductory Guide

Edited by

Cristina Camprubí, PhD

Founder and Director of GenIntegral, Barcelona
and
Assistant Professor of the Department of Cell Biology, Physiology and
Immunology of the Universitat Autònoma de Barcelona, Spain

Joan Blanco, PhD

Senior Scientist of the Genetics of Male Fertility Group
of the Universitat Autònoma de Barcelona
and
Associate Professor of the Department of Cell Biology, Physiology
and Immunology of the Universitat Autònoma de Barcelona, Spain

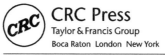

CRC Press
Taylor & Francis Group
Boca Raton London New York

CRC Press is an imprint of the
Taylor & Francis Group, an **informa** business

CRC Press
Taylor & Francis Group
6000 Broken Sound Parkway NW, Suite 300
Boca Raton, FL 33487-2742

International Standard Book Number-13: 978-1-138-63309-4 (Hardback)
978-1-138-63163-2 (Paperback)

Library of Congress Cataloging-in-Publication Data

Names: Camprubi, Cristina, editor. | Blanco, Joan, editor.
Title: Epigenetics and assisted reproduction : an introductory guide / edited by Cristina Camprubi, and Joan Blanco.
Description: Boca Raton, FL : CRC Press/Taylor & Francis Group, [2019] | Includes bibliographical references and index.
Identifiers: LCCN 2018013761| ISBN 9781138633094 (hardback : alk. paper) | ISBN 9781138631632 (paperback : alk. paper) | ISBN 9781315208701 (ebook)
Subjects: | MESH: Epigenesis, Genetic | Reproductive Techniques, Assisted | Epigenomics
Classification: LCC QH450 | NLM QU 475 | DDC 616/.042--dc23
LC record available at https://lccn.loc.gov/2018013761

Visit the Taylor & Francis Web site at
http://www.taylorandfrancis.com

and the CRC Press Web site at
http://www.crcpress.com

Contents

Preface

H UMAN FERTILITY DEPENDS ON a highly orchestrated action of hundreds of genes playing together to allow the development of highly complex mechanisms such as gametogenesis and embryogenesis. Abnormal expression of genes involved in these mechanisms has been associated to infertility affecting the assisted reproduction outcome of the affected couples. Alteration of gene expression could be caused by genetic alterations but also by epigenetic causes, which refers to heritable changes in gene expression that occur without modifications at the DNA sequence level. As contemporary medicine increasingly aims to personalize the medical approach to a patient's (epi)genetic profile, the factors that can affect gene expression also increase in importance and relevance to the clinician.

In the field of Reproductive Medicine, there is growing evidence about the influence of epigenetics on the reproductive availably of couples to conceive *in vitro*. The first evidence came from the early 2000s, when it was proved that the risk for imprinting disorders is higher in assisted reproduction technology (ART) couples. Since then, the concern of the clinicians, along with the methodological advances for the study of the epigenome, have increased our knowledge about the causes and the consequences of epigenetic variations of gametes and embryos and their effect in the ART outcome.

This handbook has been organized to provide the reader with the clues to understand the association between epigenetic variations and infertility. The first chapters introduce the main epigenetic mechanisms, followed by an extensive review of how epigenome variations of gametes and embryos are related to human infertility. We have also provided an ethical view of epigenetic variations, and an analysis about where we are and where we go from here in this field. Overall, this text will give the clinician in Reproductive Medicine a reliable grounding in current thinking and research on this fast-moving topic.

We would like to thank the book's contributors for their cooperation in putting together this excellent text. All of them are recognized scientists in their corresponding areas, and have provided valuable responses in a complex, changing, and challenging field.

Contributors

Ester Anton
Genetics of Male Fertility Group
Unitat de Biologia Cel·lular (Facultat de
    Biociències)
Universitat Autònoma de Barcelona
Cerdanyola del Vallès, Spain

Noelia Fonseca Balvís
Dpto. de Reproducción Animal
INIA
Madrid, Spain

Joan Blanco
Genetics of Male Fertility Group
Department of Cell Biology, Physiology
    and Immunology
Universitat Autònoma de Barcelona
Bellaterra (Cerdanyola del Vallès), Spain

Cristina Camprubí
GenIntegral
Barcelona
and
Department of Cell Biology, Physiology
    and Immunology
Universitat Autònoma de Barcelona
Bellaterra (Cerdanyola del Vallès), Spain

Sebastian Canovas
Department of Physiology
IMIB–Arrixaca
Regional Campus of International
    Excellence "Campus Mare Nostrum"
    University of Murcia
Murcia, Spain

Susana M. Chuva de Sousa Lopes
Department of Reproductive
    Medicine
Ghent University Hospital
Ghent, Belgium

and

Department of Anatomy and
    Embryology
Leiden University Medical
    Center
Leiden, The Netherlands

Celia Corral-Vazquez
Genetics of Male Fertility Group
Unitat de Biologia Cel·lular
    (Facultat de Biociències)
Universitat Autònoma de Barcelona
    Cerdanyola del Vallès, Spain

Pilar Coy
Department of Physiology
IMIB–Arrixaca
Regional Campus of International
    Excellence "Campus Mare Nostrum"
    University of Murcia
Murcia, Spain

Thomas Eggermann
Institute of Human Genetics
RWTH Aachen University
Aachen, Germany

Patricia Fauque
Université Bourgogne Franche-Comté-
    Equipe Génétique des Anomalies du
    Développement (GAD)
and
CHU Dijon Bourgogne
Laboratoire de Biologie de la Reproduction
Dijon, France

Raul Fernández-González
Dpto. de Reproducción Animal
INIA
Madrid, Spain

Isabel Gómez-Redondo
Dpto. de Reproducción Animal
INIA
Madrid, Spain

Carlos Guerrero-Bosagna
Avian Behavioral Genomics and
    Physiology Group
Department of Physics
and
Chemistry and Biology
Linköping University
Linköping, Sweden

Alfonso Gutiérrez-Adán
Dpto. de Reproducción Animal
INIA
Madrid, Spain

Gavin Kelsey
The Babraham Institute
Cambridge, United Kingdom

Ricardo Laguna-Barraza
Dpto. de Reproducción Animal
INIA
Madrid, Spain

Eric Marqués-García
Dpto. de Reproducción Animal
INIA
Madrid, Spain

David Monk
Imprinting and Cancer Group
Cancer Epigenetics and Biology Program
    Institut d'Investigació Biomedica de
    Bellvitge
L'Hospitalet de Llobregat
Barcelona, Spain

Ivan Nalvarte
Department of Biosciences and Nutrition
Karolinska Institutet
Huddinge, Sweden

Serafín Pérez-Cerezales
Dpto. de Reproducción Animal
INIA
Madrid, Spain

Eva Pericuesta
Dpto. de Reproducción Animal
INIA
Madrid, Spain

Benjamín Planells
Dpto. de Reproducción Animal
INIA
Madrid, Spain

George Rasti
Chromatin Biology Laboratory
Cancer Epigenetics and Biology Program
  (PEBC)
Bellvitge Biomedical Research Institute
  (IDIBELL)
L'Hospitalet de Llobregat
Barcelona, Spain

Joëlle Rüegg
Department of Clinical Neurosciences
Karolinska Institutet
Stockholm
and
Unit of Toxicology Sciences
Swetox Karolinska Institutet
Södertälje, Sweden

Josep Santaló
Universitat Autònoma de Barcelona
Unitat de Biologia Cel·lular
Facultat Biociències
Campus UAB
Bellaterra, Spain

Jörg Tost
Laboratory for Epigenetics & Environment
Centre National de Recherche en
  Génomique Humaine
CEA–Institut de Biologie Francois Jacob
Evry, France

Alejandro Vaquero
Chromatin Biology Laboratory
Cancer Epigenetics and Biology Program
  (PEBC)
Bellvitge Biomedical Research Institute
  (IDIBELL)
L'Hospitalet de Llobregat
Barcelona, Spain

CHAPTER 1

A Short Introduction to DNA Methylation

Jörg Tost

CONTENTS

1.1 INTRODUCTION

Almost all cells on an organism share the same genetic material encoded in the DNA sequence, but display a broad range of morphological and functional diversity. Epigenetics can be defined as the study of changes of a phenotype such as the gene expression patterns of a specific cell type not caused by underlying changes in the primary DNA sequence. These changes are mitotically and maybe in some cases meiotically heritable. Epigenetic regulation mediates genomic adaption to an environment thereby ultimately contributing toward the phenotype and "brings the phenotype into being" (1).

Epigenetics consists of a variety of molecular mechanisms including post-transcriptional histone modifications, histone variants, ATP-dependent chromatin remodeling complexes, polycomb/trithorax protein complexes, small and other non-coding RNAs including siRNA and miRNAs, and DNA methylation. These diverse molecular mechanisms have all been found to be closely intertwined and stabilize each other to ensure the faithful propagation of an epigenetic state over time and especially through cell division. Nonetheless epigenetic states are not static, but change with age in a stochastic manner as well as in response to environmental stimuli. This review gives a brief introduction to the multiple biological facets of DNA methylation, probably the best-studied epigenetic modification, and its potential use in clinical applications.

1.2 PATTERNS OF DNA METHYLATION

DNA methylation is a post-replication modification almost exclusively found on the 5 position of the pyrimidine ring of cytosines, (Figure 1.1), in the context of the dinucleotide sequence CpG, of which around 29 million are found in the human (haploid) genome (2). The additional methyl group is located at the major groove edge in a DNA double helix

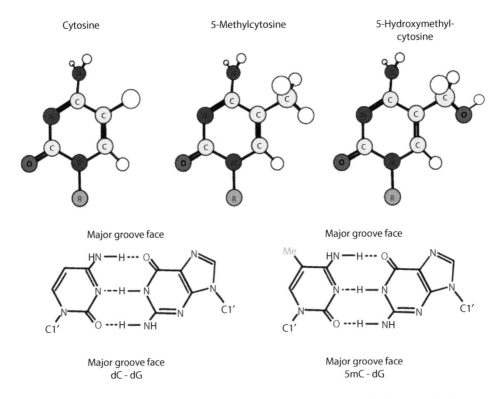

FIGURE 1.1 Chemical structure of cytosine, 5-methylcytosine, and 5-hydroxymethylcytosine. R denotes the sugar moiety, which has been omitted for simplification. Cytosine is incorporated into the DNA using deoxycytidinetriphosphate as a building block and methylated after its incorporation by DNA methyltransferases. 5-hydroxymethylcytosine is created by oxidation of methylcytosine by the TET enzymes. DNA methylation standing out in the major grove of the DNA double helix shows identical Watson-Crick base pairing compared to cytosine.

and does not change the Watson-Crick base pairing (Figure 1.1). 5-methylcytosine (5mC) accounts for ~1% of all bases, varying slightly in different tissue types and the majority (60%–80%) of CpG dinucleotides throughout mammalian genomes are methylated (Figure 1.2). Other types of methylation such as methylation of cytosines in the context of CpNpG or CpA sequences have been detected in mouse embryonic stem cells, neurons, and plants, but are generally rare in somatic mammalian/human tissues. DNA methylation marks are part of the cellular identity and memory and the sequence symmetry of CpG dinucleotides allows for the transmission of DNA methylation marks through cell division. CpGs are underrepresented in the genome, as a result of their increased mutation potential with mutation rates at CpG sites to be about 10–50 times higher than other transitional

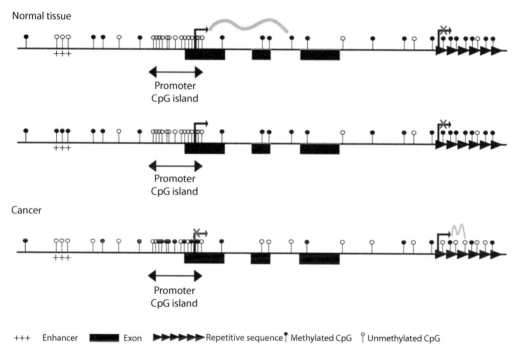

FIGURE 1.2 Distribution of DNA methylation in normal tissue and cancer. In the normal tissue, most promoter CpG islands are free of DNA methylation (indicated by white circles) even if the gene is not expressed. Repetitive elements as well as interspersed CpG dinucleotides are mostly methylated (indicated by black circles). Methylation changes at intergenic gene regulatory regions, such as enhancers, which can change the expression status of the associated gene while the methylation status of the gene does not change. In tumors, a global loss of DNA methylation (hypomethylation of the cancer genome) is observed while some promoter CpG islands become methylated in a tumor-type specific manner. Methylation patterns are dynamic and also change to a lesser extent compared to cancer with age and in response to environmental factors.

mutations. As the deamination of methylated CpGs to TpGs yields a naturally occurring DNA base, it is less well corrected. Despite this general trend, relatively CpG rich clusters, so-called CpG islands, are found in the promoter region and first exons of ∼65% genes containing about 7% of all CpGs (Figure 1.2) (3). Depending on the employed set of parameters, a CpG island is defined as having a C + G content of more than 50% (55%), an observed versus expected ratio for the occurrence of CpGs of more than 0.6 (0.65) and a minimum size of 200 (500) base pairs (4). They are mostly non-methylated in all tissues and throughout all developmental stages corresponding to an open chromatin structure and a potentially active state of transcription (Figure 1.2). There are around 30,000 CpG islands in the human genome. As CpG islands are mainly unmethylated in the germline, they are less susceptible to deamination and have therefore retained the expected frequency of CpGs. Binding of transcription factors, exclusion of nucleosomes, and the presence of H3K4 methylation and the associated histone methyltransferases protect most CpG islands from DNA methylation. It should be noted that a number of CpG islands have been identified that are methylated in a tissue-specific manner in normal tissues, but concern mainly intragenic CpG islands (5,6). CpGs islands associated to genes not expressed in a specific cell type acquire the repressive histone modification H3K27Me$_3$, but rarely DNA methylation. In contrast, regions located up- and downstream of CpG islands, termed CpG island shores, show variable tissue-specific DNA methylation patterns and these are often altered in tumorigenesis (7). In contrast to CpG islands, gene bodies are commonly highly methylated, where DNA methylation has been associated with enhanced gene expression maybe by facilitating transcriptional elongation and preventing initiation of spurious transcription events (8). Intragenic methylation has in addition been associated with the repression/use of alternative promoters or different splice variants (6,9).

1.3 DNA METHYLTRANSFERASES

Both local and global epigenetic patterns are dictated by the composition of the genome depending on CpG spacing as well as sequence motifs and DNA structure (10), while in turn DNA methylation will have a major influence on DNA shape (11). The transfer of a methyl-group from the universal methyl donor S-adenosyl-L-methionine (SAMe) is carried out by DNA methyltransferases. During the methylation reaction a methyl group is transferred from SAMe to the cytosine, thereby leaving S-adenosylhomocysteine, which at high concentrations inhibits the action of DNA methyltransferases.

Four DNA methyltransferases have been identified (*DNMT1, DNMT3A, DNMT3B,* and *DNMT3L*) (Figure 1.3) (12). DNMT3L, however, lacks a catalytic domain, but is in complex with DNMT3A important for maternal genomic imprinting and male spermatogenesis.

Simplified, DNMT1 acts as a maintenance methyltransferase as it prefers hemi-methylated templates. It is located at the replication fork during the S phase of the cell

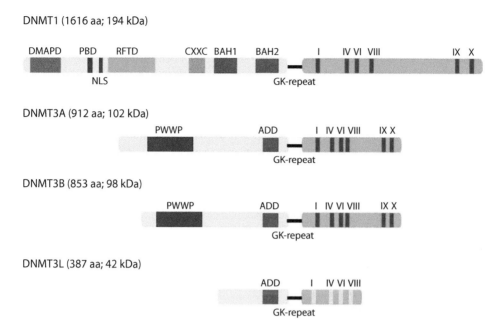

FIGURE 1.3 Schematic illustration of the domain structure of the mammalian DNMTs. All DNMTs with the exception of DNMT3L contain a catalytic domain with 10 motifs characteristic for DNA methylation activity. The DMAPD domain of DNMT1 binds DNMAP1, a factor repressing transcription through interactions with HDACs. The proliferating cell nuclear antigen (PCNA) binding domain, binds to the PBD of DNMT1, which recruits DNMT1 to replication foci at the early and middle stage of the S-phase and binds a number of factors required for replication. The RFTD domain localizes DNMT1 to the region undergoing replication by interacting with UHRF1, which recognizes hemimethylated CpGs. The CXXC domain contains two zinc atoms forming zinc fingers, which bind unmethylated CpGs. However, the exact function of this domain is currently unclear. The two BAH domains are involved in chromatin remodeling, but their exact function needs further investigation. The PWWP domain of DNMT3A and 3B is involved in protein-protein interactions, tethers the DNMTs to chromatin regions including pericentromeric heterochromatin regions marked with $H3K26Me_3$. The cysteine-rich plant homeodomain (PHD)-like ADD domain interacts with a multitude of proteins including H3K9 methylases, co-repressors, and heterochromatin protein 1. DNMT3A and 3B interact with the C-terminal domain of DNMT3L increasing *de novo* DNA methylation activity. Abbreviations used: DMAPD: DNA methyltransferase-associated protein 1 interacting domain; PBD: PCNA-binding domain; NLS: Nuclear localization signal; RFTD: Replication foci targeting domain; CXXC: CXXC domain; BAH1/2: Bromo-adjacent homology domain 1 and 2; GK-repeats: Glycine-lysine rich repeats; PWWP: PWWP domain; ADD: ATRX-DNMT3-DNMT3L domain.

cycle and methylates the newly synthesized DNA strand using the parent strand as a template with high fidelity (13). The symmetric sequence of CpGs thus allows to pass the epigenetic information to pass through cell generations. A number of proteins associated with the local chromatin structure such as LSD1 and URHF1 are required to ensure the specificity and stability of the DNA methylation reaction associated with DNA replication. However, DNMT3A and DNMT3B are also required for methylation maintenance (14). *De novo* methylation is carried out by the methyltransferases DNMT3A and DNMT3B. These enzymes have certain preferences for specific targets (e.g., DNMT3A together with DNMT3L methylates maternal imprinted genes and DNMT3B localizes at minor satellite repeats as well as the gene bodies of actively transcribed genes), but also work cooperatively to methylate the genome (12,15). Possible trigger mechanisms to initiate *de novo* methylation include preferred target DNA sequences, RNA interference, but mostly chromatin structures induced by histone modifications and other protein-protein interactions (16,17). Histone modifications such as H3K9Me$_3$ are thought to initiate heterochromatin formation and DNA methylation comes in as a secondary molecular alteration to ensure the stable silencing of the repressed sequences.

1.4 5-HYDROXYMETHYLATION AND THE DNA DEMETHYLATION PROCESSES

Mechanisms for DNA demethylation mechanism have long been searched for as active demethylation occurs at different stages of development and a global hypomethylation is associated with many cancers. DNA demethylation has been proposed to be either passive, where the 5mC is removed owing to a lack of maintaining the methylation during several cycles of replication, or as an active process, with direct removal of the methyl group independently of DNA replication (18). The active process is initiated through the enzymatic oxidation of 5mC to 5-hydroxymethylcytosine (5hmC) (Figure 1.1) as described below in this paragraph. However, 5hmC is now considered to be not only an intermediate in oxidative DNA demethylation, but constitutes a distinct layer in the complex process of epigenetic regulation with its own distribution and regulatory functions. The reaction yielding 5hmC is catalyzed by the ten-eleven translocation (TET) methylcytosine dioxygenase family of enzymes, consisting of three mammalian subtypes, TET1-3 (Figure 1.4) (12,19). 5hmC is most abundant in human brain tissue and embryonic stem cells, but at levels approximately tenfold lower than those of 5-methylcytosine (20). TET enzymes are expressed in a tissue/cell-type and developmental stage dependent manner with 5hmC decreasing during cell differentiation. Active demethylation of gene regulatory sequences plays a key role in activating specific genes required for proper tissue-specific gene expression programs. 5hmC levels do not correlate with 5mC levels of the respective tissue and 5hmC was found enriched at specific active functional elements of the genome, in particular enhancers, promoters, and

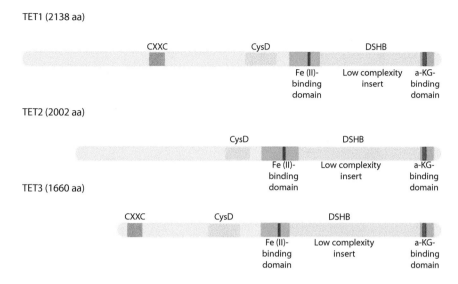

FIGURE 1.4 Domain structure of the mammalian TETs. The N-terminal region is involved in chromatin remodeling and methylation sensing and can directly bind to DNA, while the C-terminal catalytic domain consisting of a cysteine-rich domain and the double-stranded β-helix dioxygenase domain, including an Fe(II)-binding HxD motif and an α-ketoglutarate-binding domain separated by a low complexity spacer of unknown function, recognizes CpGs and oxidizes them. For TET2 the N-terminal domain is provided by a separate protein (IDAX).

gene bodies associating 5hmC with open chromatin and transcriptional activity (20,21). 5hmC levels are globally reduced in cancer and alterations of the TET enzymes have been reported for various cancers (19,22). This observation suggests that 5hmC alterations may have a distinct role in the development and progression of malignancies.

In addition to its regulatory function, 5hmC is an intermediate in the active demethylation process (23), where it is further oxidized to 5-formylcytosine (5fC) and 5-carboxylcytosine (5caC) again by the TET enzymes, with the latter two modifications being present at barely detectable levels in the human genome (Figure 1.5). Both the carboxyl and the formyl groups can be removed enzymatically with or without base excision, generating an unmethylated cytosine.

1.5 TRANSCRIPTION AND GENOME STABILITY

Transcription does not occur on naked DNA but in the context of chromatin, which critically influences the accessibility of the DNA to transcription factors and the DNA polymerase complexes. DNA methylation, histone modifications and chromatin remodeling are closely linked and constitute multiple layers of epigenetic modifications to control and modulate gene expression through chromatin structure. DNMTs and histone

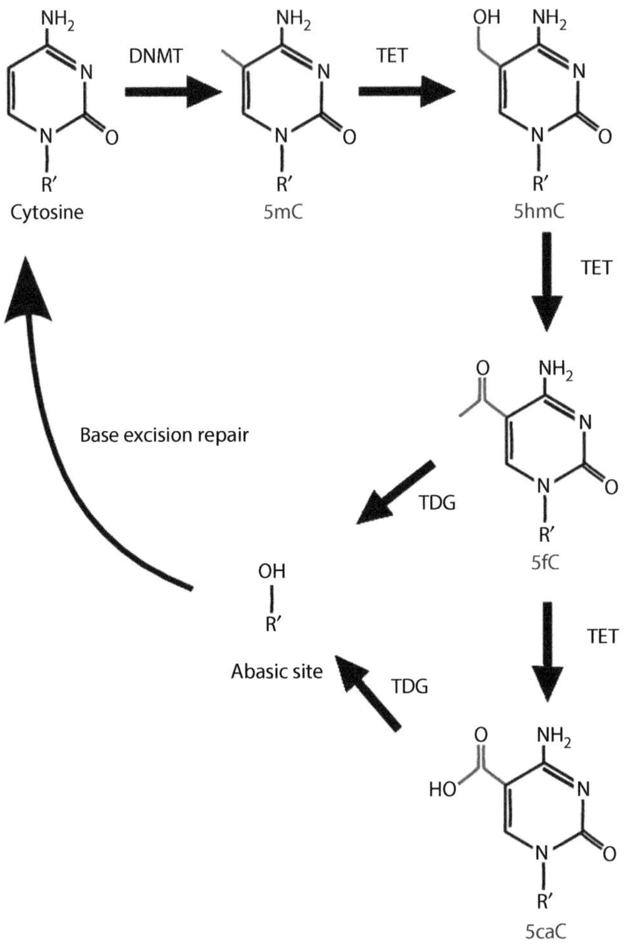

FIGURE 1.5 Demethylation pathway. TET enzymes successively oxidize 5mC to 5hmc, and 5-formylcytosine (5fC) and 5-carboxylcytosine (5caC) are dependent on α-ketoglutarate and Fe(II). 5fC and 5caC are replaced by unmodified cytosines through a thymine DNA glycosylase (TDG) initiated base excision repair (BER) mechanism, although additional mechanisms for DNA demethylation do exist.

deacetylases (HDACs) are found in the same multi-protein complexes and methyl CpG-binding domain proteins (MBDs) interact with HDACs, histone methyltransferases as well as with the chromatin remodeling complexes. Furthermore, mutations or loss of members of the SNF2 helicase/ATPase family of chromatin remodeling proteins such as ATRX or LSH lead to genome-wide perturbations of DNA methylation patterns and inappropriate gene expression programs.

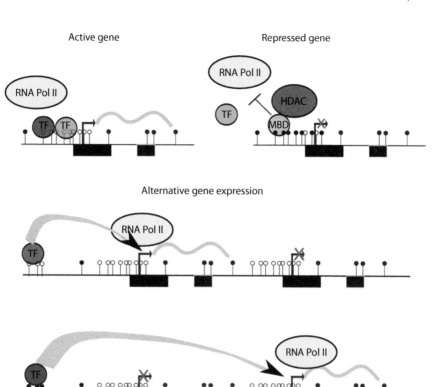

FIGURE 1.6   Methylation sensitivity of transcription factors. A simplified view how DNA methylation might influence transcription factor (TF) binding. Some TFs are only binding to unmethylated DNA and methylation will impede binding. Methylation will on the other hand attract methyl binding proteins which in complex with HDACS and other repressors will silence gene expression. Other transcription factors might also have a higher affinity for methylated compared to unmethylated DNA. Methylation changes at upstream regulatory elements such as enhancers might induce changes in the TF occupancy of the regulatory element, which can lead to activation of alternative genes or transcripts.

Transcription may be affected by DNA methylation in several ways (Figure 1.6). First, the binding of transcriptional activators such as Sp1 and Myc may be inhibited directly by the methylated DNA through sterical hindrance, while other transcription factors especially homeodomain transcription factors are attracted by methylated target recognition sequences (24–26). Methylation of CpG sites in a target sequence can thereby lead to change in transcription factor occupancy at the same sequence and activation of tissue-specific genes (27). Second, methylated DNA is bound by specific methyl-CpG binding domain (MBD1, MBD2, and MBD4) proteins or methyl-CpG binding proteins (MeCP2) as well as proteins of the Kaiso family (12,28,29). They recruit transcriptional co-repressors such as histone deacetylating complexes, polycomb proteins and chromatin remodeling complexes, thereby establishing a repressive closed chromatin configuration (Figure 1.6). Mbd3 binds specifically hydroxymethylated cytosines.

In many cases, DNA methylation occurs subsequently to changes in the chromatin structure and is used as a molecular mechanism to permanently and thus heritably lock the gene in its inactive state. It should be underlined that an unmethylated state of a CpG island or gene regulatory element does not necessarily correlate with the transcriptional activity of the gene, but rather that the gene can be potentially activated. The simple presence of methylation does therefore not necessarily induce silencing of nearby genes. Only when a specific core region of the promoter that is often—but not necessarily—spanning the transcription start site becomes hypermethylated, the expression of the associated gene is modified (30). In CpG-poor intergenic gene regulatory regions DNA methylation is highly dynamic, CpG dinucleotides are mostly highly methylated, but methylation is reduced when the region or the methylated CpG is bound by transcription factors (31).

DNA methylation plays an important role in the maintenance of genome integrity by transcriptional silencing of repetitive DNA sequences and endogenous transposons (32). DNA methylation may prevent the potentially deleterious recombination events between non-allelic repeats caused by these mobile genetic elements. In addition, methylation increases the mutation rate leading to a faster divergence of identical sequences and disabling many retrotransposons.

The functional relevance of DNA methylation (and other epigenetic changes) can now be interrogated by epigenetic editing using mainly a nuclease deficient version of the Clustered Regularly Interspaced Short Palindromic Repeats (CRISPR)/CRISPR-associated protein (Cas) 9 system, which allows recruiting chromatin modifying and remodeling complexes to specific target sequences (33). The fusion of the core catalytic domain of a DNA methyltransferase (e.g., DNMT3A) or demethylase (e.g., TET1) to a modified nuclease deficient Cas9 (dCas9) has been shown to induce specific targeted epigenetic changes either locally if a promoter is targeted or more regionally if a distant gene regulatory element such as an enhancer is targeted (33–35).

1.6 EPIGENETIC CHANGES IN HEALTH AND DISEASE

Cytosine methylation is essential for normal mammalian development including X chromosome inactivation and correct setting of genomic imprinting. Epigenetics holds the promise to explain at least a part of the influences the environment has on a phenotype as described in Chapter 5 and is an integral part of aging and cellular senescence whereby the overall content of DNA methylation in the mammalian and human genome decreases with age in all tissues especially at repetitive elements (36,37). Despite its stochastic nature,

DNA methylation levels at a number of specific loci have been shown to correlate very well with lifetime (chronological) age and several DNA methylation signatures have been developed for the accurate prediction of the age through the analysis of DNA methylation patterns (36,38). Accelerated epigenetic changing has been associated with earlier all-cause mortality in later life (39), while people with exceptional longevity show a decreased epigenetic age compared to their chronological age (40).

DNA methylation and chromatin structure are strikingly altered in many complex diseases. Mutations in genes that are part of the molecular machinery responsible for correct establishment and propagation of the epigenetic modifications through development and cell division lead to the neurodevelopmental disorders such as ICF (immune deficiency, centromeric instability, and facial abnormalities, *DNMT3B*) (41) or Rett syndrome (*MeCP2*) (42), while mutations in *TET2* have been found in multiple hematological malignancies, where they probably among the earliest genetic events of the disease (43).

Cancer is by far the most studied disease with a strong epigenetic component (44,45). In tumors, a global loss of DNA methylation (hypomethylation) of the genome is observed. This hypomethylation has been suggested to initiate and propagate oncogenesis by inducing aneuploidy, genome instability, activation of retrotransposons, and transcriptional activation of oncogenes and pro-metastatic genes (46). The overall decrease in DNA methylation is accompanied by a region- and gene-specific increase of methylation (hypermethylation) of multiple CpG islands frequently associated with transcriptional silencing of the associated gene (44,45). This hypermethylation is not random as it occurs primarily at gene promoters that are targets of the polycomb repressive complex 2 (PRC2) and marked by $H3K27Me_3$ in (embryonic) stem cells and resembles the DNA methylation changes observed during aging albeit at a much greater amplitude.

While the contribution of somatic mutations to carcinogenesis has long been recognized, it has become evident that epigenetic changes leading to transcriptional silencing of tumor suppressor genes constitute an at least equally contributing mechanism (45,47). DNA methylation changes and genetic mutations co-occurring in the same tumors show different dynamics and evolve differently during tumor progression supporting the functional relevance of epigenetic changes on the phenotype of the tumor (48). Epigenetic changes occur at higher frequency compared to genetic changes and may be especially important in early-stage human neoplasia (49).

Examples for the use of DNA methylation-based biomarkers include therefore early detection with the commercial FDA-approved Epi proColon blood test being a prime example. This test analyzes the methylation profile of an intronic sequence of the *SEPT9* gene for the population-wide screening of colorectal cancer achieving a sensitivity of 50%–80% depending of the stage of the cancer and a very high specificity (>95%) (50,51). A number of DNA methylation changes have been linked to prognosis of different cancers (52). In addition to the application for early detection of cancers, the analysis of the methylation status of CpG islands can be used to characterize and classify cancers as for examples recently demonstrated for subtypes of Ewing sarcoma, which are all characterized by the same recurrent genetic alteration (53). Furthermore, as the DNA methylation patterns of distant metastases will at least partly carry the tissue-specific DNA methylation signature of the primary tumor, analysis of the DNA methylation profile of the metastases has shown to permit the identification of the tissue of the primary tumor (54). Similarly, the DNA methylation profile of cell-free DNA from plasma/serum contains the information of the tissue it is released from and allows detecting the tissue-of-origin of a cancer (55). DNA methylation changes detect tumor recurrence as well as predict and monitor patients' response and the effectiveness to a given anti-cancer therapy with the prediction of the response of patients with glioblastomas to the alkylating agent temozolomide based on the DNA methylation status of the DNA repair gene *MGMT* being the prime example (56). As DNA methylation is a non-mutational and therefore—at least in principle—a reversible modification, it can be used as point of departure for anti-neoplastic treatment by chemically induced demethylation (57). Two DNA methyltransferase inhibitors (DNMTis) (azacytidine [Vidaza] and 5-aza-deoxycytidine [decitabine, Dacogen, Decitibine]) have been approved for the treatment of several hematological malignancies (58,59). At low doses azacytidine and decitabine induce their effect through demethylation of silenced genes associated with reduced apoptosis, cell differentiation and proliferation, whereas at higher doses the main cytotoxic effect is due to DNA damage after incorporation (60). Second-generation DNMTis with improved pharmacology and lower toxicity such as the prodrug SGI-110 show high potential for the use in the treatment of several different malignancies (58). Epigenetic therapy is rapidly evolving with many combination therapies now under investigation.

The field of epigenetics of other complex diseases is still relatively young, but epigenetics may provide the missing link between the genetic susceptibility and the phenotype by mediating and modulating environmental influences. Several neuropsychiatric disorders have been linked to epigenetic changes (61). Epigenetic dysregulation in cognitive disorders such as Alzheimer's disease as well as age-related memory decline has also been reported (62,63). DNA methylation patterns are also disturbed in atherosclerosis (64), diabetes (65) as well as inflammatory, autoimmune, and allergic diseases (66,67). In a number of studies the epigenetic changes are located in the same genomic region as genetic variation previously associated with the disease (68,69). It is difficult to infer causality from most of studies, but at least in some case DNA methylation seems to mediate the effects of genetic variation to yield the phenotype.

1.7 CONCLUSION

Although our knowledge on the regulation of DNA methylation has been rapidly increasing over the last years, the gained information has mainly led to the insight that the complexity of the gene regulatory network, in which DNA methylation plays a pivotal role, had been underestimated. CpG islands, which had been the focus of research for decades, might contribute little to the plasticity of the cells necessary for cell-type specific differentiation and to cope with internal and environmental cues. New functional tools allow now for the first time to assess the functional consequences of DNA methylation changes during development and disease. Biomedical applications of DNA methylation as biomarkers for cancer and other complex diseases, but also for prenatal testing, have become routine and first assays have been approved by regulatory agencies paving the way for a more widespread acceptance and use of DNA methylation-based tests.

REFERENCES

1. Waddington CH. The epigenotype. *Endeavour.* 1942;1:18–20.
2. Lister R, Pelizzola M, Dowen RH, Hawkins RD, Hon G, Tonti-Filippini J, Nery JR et al. Human DNA methylomes at base resolution show widespread epigenomic differences. *Nature.* 2009;462:315–22.
3. Illingworth RS, Bird AP. CpG islands—"A rough guidem" *FEBS Lett.* 2009;583:1713–20.
4. Takai D, Jones PA. Comprehensive analysis of CpG islands in human chromosomes 21 and 22. *Proc Natl Acad Sci USA.* 2002;99:3740–5.
5. Shen L, Kondo Y, Guo Y, Zhang J, Zhang L, Ahmed S, Shu J, Chen X, Waterland RA, Issa JP. Genome-wide profiling of DNA methylation reveals a class of normally methylated CpG island promoters. *PLoS Genet.* 2007;3:2023–36.
6. Maunakea AK, Nagarajan RP, Bilenky M, Ballinger TJ, D'Souza C, Fouse SD, Johnson BE et al. Conserved role of intragenic DNA methylation in regulating alternative promoters. *Nature.* 2010;466:253–7.
7. Irizarry RA, Ladd-Acosta C, Wen B, Wu Z, Montano C, Onyango P, Cui H et al. The human colon cancer methylome shows similar hypo- and hypermethylation at conserved tissue-specific CpG island shores. *Nat Genet.* 2009;41:178–86.
8. Lee SM, Choi WY, Lee J, Kim YJ. The regulatory mechanisms of intragenic DNA methylation. *Epigenomics.* 2015;7:527–31.
9. Lev Maor G, Yearim A, Ast G. The alternative role of DNA methylation in splicing regulation. *Trends Genet.* 2015;31:274–80.
10. Bock C, Paulsen M, Tierling S, Mikeska T, Lengauer T, Walter J. CpG island methylation in human lymphocytes is highly correlated with DNA sequence, repeats, and predicted DNA structure. *PLoS Genet.* 2006;2:e26.
11. Rao S, Chiu TP, Kribelbauer JF, Mann RS, Bussemaker HJ, Rohs R. Systematic prediction of DNA shape changes due to CpG methylation explains epigenetic effects on protein-DNA binding. *Epigenetics Chromatin.* 2018;11:6.

12. Ludwig AK, Zhang P, Cardoso MC. Modifiers and readers of dna modifications and their impact on genome structure, expression, and stability in disease. *Front Genet.* 2016;7:115.

13. Hermann A, Goyal R, Jeltsch A. The Dnmt1 DNA-(cytosine-C5)-methyltransferase methylates DNA processively with high preference for hemimethylated target sites. *J Biol Chem.* 2004;279:48350–9.

14. Jones PA, Liang G. Rethinking how DNA methylation patterns are maintained. *Nat Rev Genet.* 2009;10:805–11.

15. Baubec T, Colombo DF, Wirbelauer C, Schmidt J, Burger L, Krebs AR, Akalin A, Schubeler D. Genomic profiling of DNA methyltransferases reveals a role for DNMT3B in genic methylation. *Nature.* 2015;520:243–7.

16. Cheng X, Blumenthal RM. Mammalian DNA methyltransferases: A structural perspective. *Structure.* 2008;16:341–50.

17. Chedin F. The DNMT3 family of mammalian *de novo* DNA methyltransferases. *Prog Mol Biol Transl Sci.* 2011;101:255–85.

18. Franchini DM, Schmitz KM, Petersen-Mahrt SK. 5-Methylcytosine DNA demethylation: More than losing a methyl group. *Annu Rev Genet.* 2012;46:419–41.

19. Tan L, Shi YG. Tet family proteins and 5-hydroxymethylcytosine in development and disease. *Development.* 2012;139:1895–902.

20. Nestor CE, Ottaviano R, Reddington J, Sproul D, Reinhardt D, Dunican D, Katz E, Dixon JM, Harrison DJ, Meehan RR. Tissue type is a major modifier of the 5-hydroxymethylcytosine content of human genes. *Genome Res.* 2012;22:467–77.

21. Ficz G, Branco MR, Seisenberger S, Santos F, Krueger F, Hore TA, Marques CJ, Andrews S, Reik W. Dynamic regulation of 5-hydroxymethylcytosine in mouse ES cells and during differentiation. *Nature.* 2011;473:398–402.

22. Putiri EL, Tiedemann RL, Thompson JJ, Liu C, Ho T, Choi JH, Robertson KD. Distinct and overlapping control of 5-methylcytosine and 5-hydroxymethylcytosine by the TET proteins in human cancer cells. *Genome Biol.* 2014;15:R81.

23. Wu SC, Zhang Y. Active DNA demethylation: Many roads lead to Rome. *Nat Rev Mol Cell Biol.* 2010;11:607–20.

24. Yin Y, Morgunova E, Jolma A, Kaasinen E, Sahu B, Khund-Sayeed S, Das PK et al. Impact of cytosine methylation on DNA binding specificities of human transcription factors. *Science.* 2017;356:eaaj2239.

25. Hu S, Wan J, Su Y, Song Q, Zeng Y, Nguyen HN, Shin J et al. DNA methylation presents distinct binding sites for human transcription factors. *eLife.* 2013;2:e00726.

26. Kribelbauer JF, Laptenko O, Chen S, Martini GD, Freed-Pastor WA, Prives C, Mann RS, Bussemaker HJ. Quantitative analysis of the DNA methylation sensitivity of transcription factor complexes. *Cell Rep.* 2017;19:2383–95.

27. Rishi V, Bhattacharya P, Chatterjee R, Rozenberg J, Zhao J, Glass K, Fitzgerald P, Vinson C. CpG methylation of half-CRE sequences creates C/EBPalpha binding sites that activate some tissue-specific genes. *Proc Natl Acad Sci USA* 2010;107:20311–6.

28. Baubec T, Ivanek R, Lienert F, Schubeler D. Methylation-dependent and -independent genomic targeting principles of the MBD protein family. *Cell.* 2013;153:480–92.

29. Shimbo T, Wade PA. Proteins that read DNA methylation. *Adv Exp Med Biol.* 2016;945:303–20.

30. Ushijima T. Detection and interpretation of altered methylation patterns in cancer cells. *Nat Rev Cancer.* 2005;5:223–31.

31. Stadler MB, Murr R, Burger L, Ivanek R, Lienert F, Scholer A, van Nimwegen E et al. DNA-binding factors shape the mouse methylome at distal regulatory regions. *Nature*. 2011;480:490–5.
32. Lippman Z, Gendrel AV, Black M, Vaughn MW, Dedhia N, McCombie WR, Lavine K et al. Role of transposable elements in heterochromatin and epigenetic control. *Nature*. 2004;430:471–6.
33. Thakore PI, Black JB, Hilton IB, Gersbach CA. Editing the epigenome: Technologies for programmable transcription and epigenetic modulation. *Nat Methods*. 2016;13:127–37.
34. Choudhury SR, Cui Y, Lubecka K, Stefanska B, Irudayaraj J. CRISPR-dCas9 mediated TET1 targeting for selective DNA demethylation at BRCA1 promoter. *Oncotarget*. 2016;7:46545–56.
35. Vojta A, Dobrinic P, Tadic V, Bockor L, Korac P, Julg B, Klasic M, Zoldos V. Repurposing the CRISPR-Cas9 system for targeted DNA methylation. *Nucleic Acids Res*. 2016;44:5615–28.
36. Hannum G, Guinney J, Zhao L, Zhang L, Hughes G, Sadda S, Klotzle B et al. Genome-wide methylation profiles reveal quantitative views of human aging rates. *Mol Cell*. 2013;49:359–67.
37. Jones MJ, Goodman SJ, Kobor MS. DNA methylation and healthy human aging. *Aging Cell*. 2015;14:924–32.
38. Horvath S. DNA methylation age of human tissues and cell types. *Genome Biol*. 2013;14:R115.
39. Marioni RE, Shah S, McRae AF, Chen BH, Colicino E, Harris SE, Gibson J et al. DNA methylation age of blood predicts all-cause mortality in later life. *Genome Biol*. 2015;16:25.
40. Armstrong NJ, Mather KA, Thalamuthu A, et al. Aging, exceptional longevity and comparisons of the Hannum and Horvath epigenetic clocks. *Epigenomics*. 2017;9:689–700.
41. Weng YL, An R, Shin J, Wright MJ, Trollor JN, Ames D, Brodaty H, Schofield PR, Sachdev PS, Kwok JB. DNA modifications and neurological disorders. *Neurotherapeutics: ASENT*. 2013;10:556–67.
42. Leonard H, Cobb S, Downs J. Clinical and biological progress over 50 years in Rett syndrome. *Nat Rev Neurol*. 2017;13:37–51.
43. Chiba S. Dysregulation of TET2 in hematologic malignancies. *Int J Hematol*. 2017;105:17–22.
44. Dawson MA, Kouzarides T. Cancer epigenetics: From mechanism to therapy. *Cell*. 2012;150:12–27.
45. Baylin SB, Jones PA. Epigenetic determinants of cancer. *Cold Spring Harb Perspect Biol*. 2016;8.
46. Ehrlich M, Lacey M. DNA hypomethylation and hemimethylation in cancer. *Adv Exp Med Biol*. 2013;754:31–56.
47. Balmain A, Gray J, Ponder B. The genetics and genomics of cancer. *Nat Genet*. 2003;33(Suppl.):238–44.
48. Li S, Garrett-Bakelman FE, Chung SS, Sanders MA, Hricik T, Rapaport F, Patel J et al. Distinct evolution and dynamics of epigenetic and genetic heterogeneity in acute myeloid leukemia. *Nat Med*. 2016;22:792–9.
49. Fleischer T, Frigessi A, Johnson KC, Edvardsen H, Touleimat N, Klajic J, Riis ML et al. Genome-wide DNA methylation profiles in progression to *in situ* and invasive carcinoma of the breast with impact on gene transcription and prognosis. *Genome Biol*. 2014;15:435.
50. Lamb YN, Dhillon S. Epi proColon® 2.0 CE: A blood-based screening test for colorectal cancer. *Mol Diagn Ther*. 2017;21:225–32.
51. Church TR, Wandell M, Lofton-Day C, Mongin SJ, Burger M, Payne SR, Castanos-Velez E et al. Prospective evaluation of methylated SEPT9 in plasma for detection of asymptomatic colorectal cancer. *Gut*. 2014;63:317–25.

52. How Kit A, Nielsen HM, Tost J. DNA methylation based biomarkers: Practical considerations and applications. *Biochimie*. 2012;94:2314–37.

53. Sheffield NC, Pierron G, Klughammer J, Datlinger P, Schonegger A, Schuster M, Hadler J et al. DNA methylation heterogeneity defines a disease spectrum in Ewing sarcoma. *Nat Med*. 2017;23:386–95.

54. Moran S, Martinez-Cardus A, Sayols S, Musulen E, Balana C, Estival-Gonzalez A, Moutinho C et al. Epigenetic profiling to classify cancer of unknown primary: A multicentre, retrospective analysis. *Lancet Oncol*. 2016;17:1386–95.

55. Guo S, Diep D, Plongthongkum N, Fung HL, Zhang K, Zhang K. Identification of methylation haplotype blocks aids in deconvolution of heterogeneous tissue samples and tumor tissue-of-origin mapping from plasma DNA. *Nat Genet*. 2017;49:635–42.

56. Hegi ME, Diserens AC, Gorlia T, Hamou MF, de Tribolet N, Weller M, Kros JM et al. MGMT gene silencing and benefit from temozolomide in glioblastoma. *N Engl J Med*. 2005;352:997–1003.

57. Ahuja N, Easwaran H, Baylin SB. Harnessing the potential of epigenetic therapy to target solid tumors. *J Clin Invest*. 2014;124:56–63.

58. Treppendahl MB, Kristensen LS, Gronbaek K. Predicting response to epigenetic therapy. *J Clin Invest*. 2014;124:47–55.

59. Gros C, Fahy J, Halby L, Dufau I, Erdmann A, Gregoire JM, Ausseil F, Vispe S, Arimondo PB. DNA methylation inhibitors in cancer: Recent and future approaches. *Biochimie*. 2012;94:2280–96.

60. Gnyszka A, Jastrzebski Z, Flis S. DNA methyltransferase inhibitors and their emerging role in epigenetic therapy of cancer. *Anticancer Res*. 2013;33:2989–96.

61. Ai S, Shen L, Guo J, Feng X, Tang B. DNA methylation as a biomarker for neuropsychiatric diseases. *Int J Neurosci*. 2012;122:165–76.

62. Day JJ, Sweatt JD. Epigenetic mechanisms in cognition. *Neuron*. 2011;70:813–29.

63. Smith RG, Lunnon K. DNA modifications and Alzheimer's disease. *Adv Exp Med Biol*. 2017;978:303–19.

64. Valencia-Morales Mdel P, Zaina S, Heyn H, Carmona FJ, Varol N, Sayols S, Condom E et al. The DNA methylation drift of the atherosclerotic aorta increases with lesion progression. *BMC Med Genomics*. 2015;8:7.

65. Ronn T, Ling C. DNA methylation as a diagnostic and therapeutic target in the battle against Type 2 diabetes. *Epigenomics*. 2015;7:451–60.

66. Fogel O, Richard-Miceli C, Tost J. Epigenetic changes in chronic inflammatory diseases. *Adv Protein Chem Struct Biol*. 2017;106:139–89.

67. Potaczek DP, Harb H, Michel S, Alhamwe BA, Renz H, Tost J. Epigenetics and allergy: From basic mechanisms to clinical applications. *Epigenomics*. 2017;9:539–71.

68. Liu Y, Aryee MJ, Padyukov L, Fallin MD, Hesselberg E, Runarsson A, Reinius L et al. Epigenome-wide association data implicate DNA methylation as an intermediary of genetic risk in rheumatoid arthritis. *Nat Biotechnol*. 2013;31:142–7.

69. Low D, Mizoguchi A, Mizoguchi E. DNA methylation in inflammatory bowel disease and beyond. *World J Gastroenterol*. 2013;19:5238–49.

CHAPTER 2

Epigenetic Modifications of Histones

George Rasti and Alejandro Vaquero

CONTENTS

2.1 INTRODUCTION

In eukaryotic cells, nuclear DNA is organized with histones into chromatin to allow the dynamic and efficient regulation of its functions. Chromatin is regulated to a great extent by epigenetic information, which not only determines the physical organization of the genome, but also controls access to genetic information through modulation of its structure. Much of this epigenetic information is stored in post-translational modifications (PTMs) of histones. These modifications, or marks, are involved in virtually all DNA-related functions, including genome structure and organization, gene expression, DNA replication and repair, cell cycle, and apoptosis, among others. This is reflected by the well-established effects of histone PTMs alteration on many physiological processes, such as changes in gene expression, metabolism, chromosome segregation, genome instability, and developmental abnormalities. These PTMs involve the modification of specific residues in the exposed regions of histones, mainly at the N-terminal tail, and include a wide range of chemical modifications, the most relevant of which are acetylation, methylation, phosphorylation, ubiquitination, sumoylation, and ADP-ribosylation. Histone modifications are very dynamic, since they can be added or removed by a variety of enzymes. The potential complexity of these marks is considerable as many of them target more than one type of residue and can be established in several conformations involving different numbers of these marks (1). Although some of them may play a direct structural role, they signal specific functional outputs by serving as docking sites for the binding of reader proteins that carry out this function. These marks do not act alone; they interact with each other and with the rest of the epigenetic machinery, including DNA methylation, non-coding RNA, and histone variants (2).

Alterations of these marks or the enzymes involved have dramatic effects on viability and development. They also play a major role in the maintenance of cell identity, since they regulate the transition between all differentiation steps, participate in cell stemness, and have a clear impact on cell fate (3). In this chapter, we will describe these histone modifications and discuss their links with gametogenesis, fertilization, and early development.

2.2 HISTONE MODIFICATIONS

To date, 16 histone PTMs have been described. Of them, acetylation and methylation are the best studied and most functionally relevant to the regulation of gene expression, chromatin structure, and organization (4).

Histone Acetylation

Histone acetylation occurs at lysine residues mainly located on the amino-terminal tails of histones. It is associated with increased DNA accessibility and active transcription through a dual mode of action involving a general structural effect on chromatin fiber, and by acting as docking sites for proteins containing the acetyl readers known as bromodomains. In contrast, deacetylation reduces DNA accessibility, and increases chromatin condensation, thereby promoting transcriptional repression (5). The levels of acetylation are maintained by a balance between opposing groups of enzymes: Histone acetyl transferases (HATs) and histone deacetylases (HDACs). The members of the class III HDACs, or Sirtuins, are particularly interesting as they are closely involved in the response to oxidative and genotoxic stress, which are both conditions that have been linked to defects in gametogenesis or early embryogenesis (6).

Histone Methylation

Methylation of histones occurs at lysine and arginine residues. Lysine residues can be mono-, di- or trimethylated (me1, me2, me3). Lysine methylation and demethylation are mediated by histone methyltransferases (HMTs) and histone demethylases (KDMs), respectively. Arginine methylation is catalyzed by protein arginine methyltransferases (PRMTs), and it can be dimethylated symmetrically or asymmetrically.

Unlike acetylation, methylation does not alter the histone charge and their action is mainly based on specific binding of readers. It occurs predominantly on histones H3 and H4, and may also be a marker for active or inactive chromatin regions. Transcriptionally active chromatin is characterized by high levels of lysine acetylation and by H3K4me3, H3K36me3, and H3K79me3. On the other hand, heterochromatin or compacted inactive chromatin is characterized by low levels of acetylation and high levels of H3K9me2-3, H3K27me2-3, and H4K20me3 (7–9) (Table 2.1).

TABLE 2.1   Post-Translational Histone Modifications (PTMs) Involved in Gametogenesis and Early Embriogenesis

Histone Code	Function	Implication
H2A119ub	Gene silencing	Oogenesis
H2AX Phospho	Gene silencing	Stress response
H2Bub (p21)	Gene activation	Cell cycle progression
H3K27ac	Chromatin decompaction/Active transcription	Early embryogenesis
H4K5ac	Chromatin decompaction/Active transcription	Early embryogenesis
H4K8ac	Chromatin decompaction/Active transcription	Oogenesis
H4K12ac	Chromatin decompaction/Active transcription	Oogenesis
H4K16ac	Chromatin decompaction/Active transcription	Oogenesis
H3K4me1-me3	Chromatin decompaction/Active transcription	Oogenesis/Spermatogenesis/ Early embryogenesis
H3K9me2, me3	Chromatin compaction/Gene silencing	Oogenesis/Spermatogenesis/ Early embryogenesis
H3K27me2,me3	Chromatin compaction/Gene silencing	Oogenesis/Spermatogenesis/ Early embryogenesis
H3S10 Phospho	Gene activation	Cell cycle progression
H4K20 me1-me3	Chromatin compaction/Gene silencing	Early embryogenesis
PRM (Phospho, disulfide)	Gene silencing	Spermatogenesis

Histone Phosphorylation

Histone phosphorylation is a highly dynamic mark regulated by kinases and phosphatases that respectively add and remove the phosphate groups. Histones phosphorylations are predominately related to gene activation and take place in serine, threonine, and tyrosine residues although they can also play an opposite role. For example, while phosphorylation of H3S10 is associated with activation of gene transcription, histone variant H2AX phosphorylation at Ser139 (γH2AX) correlates with DNA damage, chromosome condensation, and gene silencing (10).

Histone Ubiquitination and Sumoylation

Histones lysine residues can also be modified by addition of nine kDa proteins, the most relevant being ubiquitin. Ubiquitination associates with gene expression or repression (11). For instance, H2AK119 ubiquitination leads to polycomb-associated silencing, whereas mono-ubiquitination of histone H2B in p21 gene associates with p53-dependent transcriptional (12). Lysines can also undergo addition of SUMO1-3, ubiquitin-like proteins associated with gene activation and gene silencing (13).

Histone ADP-Ribosylation

ADP-ribosylation (ADPR) involves the addition of the ADP-ribose moiety of NAD$^+$. Some members of the PARP superfamily have been shown to promote mono- or poly-ADPR of histones. The levels of poly ADP-ribosylation, PARP-1, and PARP-2 catalytic activity (14), and the turnover of ADP-ribosyl residues all decreased during the differentiation of the germinal cell line, most noticeably at the end of spermiogenesis, which suggests a possible role for this modification in male fertility (15).

2.3 HISTONE MARKS IN HUMAN REPRODUCTION

Role in Gametogenesis

Spermatogenesis

The process of spermatogenesis involves a continuous process of germ-cell proliferation and differentiation involving DNA methylation, chromatin remodeling and condensation, and gradual replacement of histones by protamines. All these events are tightly regulated by histone PTMs, including acetylation, methylation, phosphorylation, and ubiquitination (summarized in Table 2.1). For instance, Sirtuins have been directly linked to spermatogenesis (16,17). *Sirt1$^{-/-}$* mice are more infertile, characterized by lower levels of mature sperm and spermatogenic precursors, and immotile sperm arising from the altered expression of genes related to spermatogenesis (18). Moreover, the HMTs EZH1 and EZH2, catalytic subunits of PRC2 complexes, regulate H3K27me3 during gametogenesis. Germline ablation of both EZH1 and EHZ2 in mice promotes a global depletion of H3K27me3 levels and meiotic arrest in spermatocytes (19). Additionally, lysine demethylase KDM1A/LSD1 plays an important role in spermatogenesis by reducing H3K4me2 levels (20) (Table 2.1).

Protamines interact with DNA more tightly than histones, creating a compact, toroidal structure that protects the DNA. PRM1 and PRM2, the two best-characterized protamines, undergo PTM such as phosphorylation (serine, threonine, and tyrosine residues) and disulfide bond formation. Mammalian hyperacetylated testicular histones are first replaced by transition proteins (TNPs), small proteins (50–140aa) enriched in arginine and lysine residues. Subsequently, the testis-specific histone H2B variant TH2B is loaded into spermatid chromatin by TNP1 and TNP2 (21–23). TNPs are substituted by PRM1 and PRM2, previously phosphorylated by serine/arginine protein-specific kinase 1 (SRPK1) and calcium/calmodulin-dependent protein kinase 4 (CAMK4), respectively (24,25). During spermatid elongation, protamines are dephosphorylated allowing the formation of disulfide bonds between dephosphorylated cysteine residues preventing their dislocation from DNA (26). In fertile men, the PRM1:PRM2 ratio is strictly regulated to maintain a value of approximately 1:1. The shift of this ratio has been associated with poor semen quality and male reproductive disorders. This protamine-rich chromatin makes spermatid nuclei more compact and protects sperm DNA from damage during sperm transport in the male and female reproductive tracts (27). Interestingly, the JmjC-containing histone demethylase 2a (JHDM2A) is recruited to the promoter regions of *Tnp1* and *Prm1* genes, to remove H3K9me2,3, leading to transcriptional activation of these genes (28) (Figure 2.1).

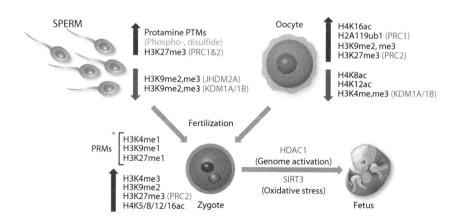

FIGURE 2.1 Main alterations of histone PTMs and related enzymes during gametogenesis, fertilization, and early embryogenesis. *Refers to PTMs of histones in sperm pronucleus that replace protamines (PRMs) as explained in the text.

Oogenesis

Oocytes remain arrested during prophase of the first meiotic division (prophase-I) for decades in humans. This prophase-I arrest is highly conserved in metazoans and is critical for oocyte differentiation because allows the oocyte to accumulate maternal components to ensure completion of oogenesis and activation of the embryonic genome upon fertilization. The oocyte contains histone-bound maternal DNA acquired during oogenesis comprising PTMs related to stalled metaphase-II. The most important difference between the chromatin of oocytes and of somatic nuclei is the absence of somatic linker histone H1 in oocytes, which is replaced with a specific histone H1 variant whose function remains elusive. Moreover, the histone H4 acetylation pattern changes during oogenesis, whereby the levels of H4K8ac and H4K12ac decrease as the oocytes mature, while that of H4K16ac increases (Figure 2.1). Interestingly, HDAC1 and 2 are important regulators of oogenesis through gene repression. While HDAC2 is essential in oocyte development, HDAC1 is more responsible for cell-cycle regulation and zygotic development (29,30). In contrast, SIRT1 deficiency does not seem to alter oocyte production in female mice (31).

Evidence also suggests that histone methylation marks such as active H3K4me3 and inactive H3K9me3 are required in follicle and oocyte meiotic maturation (32,33). In *Drosophila*, the H3K9me3 HMTs dSETDB1/Eggless, SU (VAR)3-9, and dG9a, are very important regulators of oogenesis and are critical for fertility (34). Histone H2AK119 mono-ubiquitination by the polycomb repressive complex 1 (PRC1), and H3K27me3 by PRC2, also play a key role in repression of developmental genes to maintain ES cell identity (35,36). Moreover, H3K4 demethylation is, as in the case of spermatogenesis, critical for establishing DNA methylation imprinting during oogenesis. KDM1A or KDM1B are responsible for demethylating H3K4me1,me2 during oogenesis and preimplantation embryogenesis (37) (Table 2.1).

The Role of Histone Post-Translational Modifications in Fertilization and Early Embryogenesis

Immediately after fertilization and zygote formation takes place, a rapid demethylation of DNA and histones, which is a critical process for dedifferentiated embryo formation. Both are established during gametogenesis, where they regulate gene promoters involved in gene imprinting in the embryo. However, unlike DNA methylation, histone PTMs are stable during the proliferative and meiotic phases of spermatogenesis. Interestingly, the histone marks H3K9me3 and H3K20me2 are predominately associated with methylated DNA in both embryo and placenta. These parent-of-origin-specific epigenetic changes cause differential expression of specific genes in the embryo, mainly encoding transcription and growth factors. Gene imprinting in sperm depends on the PTMs of the remaining histones, like H3K9me3 and H4K20me3 (38). The female pronucleus carries a number of active marks like H3K4me2/3, H4K8/12 ac, all of which are not altered globally during fertilization. In contrast, sperm chromatin undergoes major changes such as replacement of protamines with H3K4me1, H3K9me1, and H3K27me1 and subsequent appearance of H3K4me3, H3K9me2, H3K27me3, and acetylated form of H4K5/8/12/16 (39) (Figure 2.1 and Table 2.1). It was shown that *Suv4-20h1/h2*, the H4K20me2,3 HMTs, are mainly absent in preimplantation mouse embryos, leading to a rapid decrease of H4K20me3 from the 2-cell stage onward until the peri-implantation period (40). Other histone marks are also important in regulation of gene expression during early stages of development. After fertilization, H3K27ac progressively decreases from the early pronuclear stage to 8-cell stage, corresponding to major embryonic genome activation, followed by H3K27 re-acetylation from the morula stage onward (41). In contrast, the non-canonical H3K4me3 is subjected to massive reprogramming. This involves a massive loss from the early to the late 2-cell stage embryo, followed by a re-establishment of H3K4me3 on promoter regions, which is maintained till blastocyst stage (Figure 2.2). Meanwhile, H3K27me3 levels decrease massively from the late 2-cell stage embryo to blastocyst. The distinct features of H3K4me3 and H3K27me3 are essential for zygotic

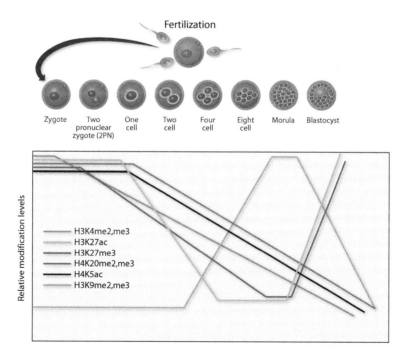

FIGURE 2.2 Dynamics of relevant histone modifications during early embryogenesis from fertilization to blastocyte.

genome activation and the further development (42). H3K9me2,me3 levels increase from the 4-cell stage and peak at morula stage, but their levels decrease again during the blastocyst stage (Figure 2.2) (43,44). HDAC1 regulates gene expression in mouse preimplantation embryos by deacetylating histone H4, and especially H4K5Ac. Sirtuins are also important in gametogenesis and early embryo development in the context of the response to metabolic and stress conditions. Thus, during post-fertilization events, maternally derived SIRT3 is essential for protecting early-stage embryos from stress conditions by inhibiting of the ROS-p53 pathway. Moreover, SIRT3 plays a protective role in mouse preimplantation embryos under *in vitro* culture conditions. Although *Sirt3*-/- mice are fertile, embryos derived from *in vitro*-cultured *Sirt3*-/- are susceptible to developmental defects (45).

2.4 THE ROLE OF PTMS IN ASSISTED REPRODUCTIVE TECHNOLOGY

Assisted reproductive technology (ART) has become a popular option for the treatment of human infertility. This technology is considered to be safe with respect to major congenital malformations and chromosomal aberrations (46). However, evidence suggests that ART, and particularly intracytoplasmic sperm injection (ICSI), may cause epigenetic alterations in the human preimplantation embryo, including higher rates of *de novo* sex chromosomal aberrations (CAs), microdeletions, polymorphisms, and spermatozoan aneuploidy (47). This may be due in part to the *in vitro* manipulation of the gametes and the preimplantation embryos inducing an adaptive response that, in turn, alters the epigenetic information. These conditions can also enhance oxidative or genotoxic stress, which may be potentially responsible for the low efficiency of fertilization by ATRs (48). Although this association was first established related to DNA methylation in imprinting disorders (49), a growing body of evidence has identified a correlation between ART and changes in histone marks. For instance, *in vitro* maturation altered histone acetylation and deacetylation activity in oocytes, leading to reduced expression of HDAC1 and of the HAT GCN5 in oocytes (50). Treatment of class I-II HDAC inhibitor TSA after SCNT in bovine embryos seems to affect the cell number of the inner cell mass of the resulting blastocysts and substantially improve the preimplantation development of cloned bovine embryos (51,52). Mouse oocytes subjected to vitrification consistently showed higher levels of H3K9me2,3 H4K5ac, and H4K12ac (53), whereas oocytes matured *in vitro* contain lowered levels of H4K16ac (50). Other studies in mice showed that although the pattern of H3K4me3 of *in vivo* and IVF embryos was similar from zygote to blastocyst stages, they were significantly lower in the mouse preimplantation embryos from meiosis-II oocytes fertilized *in vitro* compared with *in vivo* embryos. Notably, TSA treatment partially rescued levels of H3K4me3 in these embryos (54).

2.5 CONCLUDING REMARKS AND PERSPECTIVES

Evidence suggests an important role of histone PTMs in gametogenesis, fertilization, and early embryonic development. The main methods for assessing sperm, oocyte, and embryo quality in ART are currently based on morphological analysis and do not take these PTMs into account. Thus, the analysis of specific modifications or combinations of them, could identify biomarkers o predict fertility efficiency and to evaluate the risks associated with particular fertilized embryos. Some epigenetic biomarkers of fertility have already been validated or are currently under study (55,56). Establishing links between epigenetic errors in both offspring and parents and the methods of ART used could help determine the impact of each particular technique on the embryo epigenome.

REFERENCES

1. Peterson CL, Laniel M-A. Histones and histone modifications. *Curr Biol.* 2004;14:R546–51.
2. Kouzarides T. SnapShot: Histone-modifying enzymes. *Cell.* 2007;131.
3. Cantone I, Fisher AG. Epigenetic programming and reprogramming during development. *Nat Struct Mol Biol.* 2013;20:282–9.
4. Rando OJ. Combinatorial complexity in chromatin structure and function: Revisiting the histone code. *Curr Opin Genet Dev.* 2012;22:148–55.
5. Clayton AL, Hazzalin CA, Mahadevan LC. Enhanced histone acetylation and transcription: A dynamic perspective. *Mol Cell.* 2006;23:289–96.
6. Kuo MH, Allis CD. Roles of histone acetyltransferases and deacetylases in gene regulation. *BioEssays.* 1998;20:615–26.
7. Bannister AJ, Kouzarides T. Regulation of chromatin by histone modifications. *Cell Res.* 2011;21:381–95.
8. Rea S, Eisenhaber F, O'Carroll D et al. Regulation of chromatin structure by site-specific histone H3 methyltransferases. *Nature.* 2000;406(6796):593–9.
9. Hublitz P, Albert M, Peters AHFM. Mechanisms of transcriptional repression by histone lysine methylation. *Int J Dev Biol [Internet].* 2009;53(2–3):335–54. Available from: http://www.ncbi.nlm.nih.gov/pubmed/19412890
10. Rossetto D, Avvakumov N, Côté J. Histone phosphorylation: A chromatin modification involved in diverse nuclear events. *Epigenetics.* 2012;7:1098–108.
11. Cao J, Yan Q. Histone ubiquitination and deubiquitination in transcription, DNA damage response, and cancer. *Front Oncol [Internet].* 2012;2, Available from: http://journal.frontiersin.org/article/10.3389/fonc.2012.00026/abstract
12. Minsky N, Shema E, Field Y, Schuster M, Segal E, Oren M. Monoubiquitinated H2B is associated with the transcribed region of highly expressed genes in human cells. *Nat Cell Biol.* 2008;10(4):483–8.
13. Shen Z, Pardington-Purtymun PE, Comeaux JC, Moyzis RK, Chen DJ. UBL1, a human ubiquitin-like protein associating with human RAD51/RAD52 proteins. *Genomics [Internet].* 1996;36(2):271–9. Available from: http://linkinghub.elsevier.com/retrieve/pii/S0888754396904620

14. Martinez-Zamudio R, Ha HC. Histone ADP-ribosylation facilitates gene transcription by directly remodeling nucleosomes. *Mol Cell Biol [Internet]*. 2012;32(13):2490–502. Available from: http://mcb.asm.org/cgi/doi/10.1128/MCB.06667-11

15. Schrick JJ, Vogel P, Abuin A, Hampton B, Rice DS. ADP-ribosylation factor-like 3 is involved in kidney and photoreceptor development. *Am J Pathol [Internet]*. 2006;168(4):1288–98. Available from: http://www.pubmedcentral.nih.gov/articlerender.fcgi?artid=1606550&tool=pmcentrez&rendertype=abstract

16. Surani MA, Hayashi K, Hajkova P. Genetic and epigenetic regulators of pluripotency. *Cell*. 2007;128:747–62.

17. Kimmins S, Sassone-Corsi P. Chromatin remodelling and epigenetic features of germ cells. *Nature*. 2005;434:583–9.

18. McBurney MW, Yang X, Jardine K et al. The mammalian SIR2alpha protein has a role in embryogenesis and gametogenesis. *Mol Cell Biol [Internet]*. 2003;23(1):38–54. Available from: http://www.pubmedcentral.nih.gov/articlerender.fcgi?artid=140671&tool=pmcentrez&rendertype=abstract

19. Mu W, Starmer J, Shibata Y, Yee D, Magnuson T. EZH1 in germ cells safeguards the function of PRC2 during spermatogenesis. *Dev Biol*. 2017;424(2):198–207.

20. Siklenka K, Erkek S, Godmann M et al. Disruption of histone methylation in developing sperm impairs offspring health transgenerationally. *Science (80-) [Internet]*. 2015;350(6261):aab2006–aab2006. Available from: http://www.sciencemag.org/cgi/doi/10.1126/science.aab2006

21. Montellier E, Boussouar F, Rousseaux S et al. Chromatin-to-nucleoprotamine transition is controlled by the histone H2B variant TH2B. *Genes Dev*. 2013;27(15):1680–92.

22. Balhorn R, Brewer L, Corzett M. DNA condensation by protamine and arginine-rich peptides: Analysis of toroid stability using single DNA molecules. *Mol Reprod Dev*. 2000;56(2 Suppl.):230–4.

23. Fuentes-Mascorro G, Serrano H, Rosado A. Sperm chromatin. *Arch Androl*. 2000;45(3):215–25.

24. Papoutsopoulou S, Nikolakaki E, Chalepakis G, Kruft V, Chevaillier P, Giannakouros T. SR protein-specific kinase 1 is highly expressed in testis and phosphorylates protamine 1. *Nucleic Acids Res*. 1999;27(14):2972–80.

25. Wu JY, Ribar TJ, Cummings DE, Burton KA, McKnight GS, Means AR. Spermiogenesis and exchange of basic nuclear proteins are impaired in male germ cells lacking Camk4. *Nat Genet*. 2000;25(4):448–52.

26. Vilfan ID, Conwell CC, Hud NV. Formation of native-like mammalian sperm cell chromatin with folded bull protamine. *J Biol Chem*. 2004;279(19):20088–95.

27. Gazquez C, Oriola J, de Mateo S, Vidal-Taboada JM, Ballesca JL, Oliva R. A common protamine 1 promoter polymorphism (–190 C→A) correlates with abnormal sperm morphology and increased protamine P1/P2 ratio in infertile patients. *J Androl [Internet]*. 2008;29(5):540–8. Available from: http://doi.wiley.com/10.2164/jandrol.107.004390

28. Okada Y, Scott G, Ray MK, Mishina Y, Zhang Y. Histone demethylase JHDM2A is critical for Tnp1 and Prm1 transcription and spermatogenesis. *Nature*. 2007;450(7166):119–23.

29. Ma P, de Waal E, Weaver JR, Bartolomei MS, Schultz RM. A DNMT3A2-HDAC2 complex is essential for genomic imprinting and genome integrity in mouse oocytes. *Cell Rep*. 2015;13(8):1552–60.

30. Ma P, Schultz RM. HDAC1 and HDAC2 in mouse oocytes and preimplantation embryos: Specificity versus compensation. *Cell Death Differ*. 2016;23:1119–27.

31. Coussens M, Maresh JG, Yanagimachi R, Maeda G, Allsopp R. *Sirt1* deficiency attenuates spermatogenesis and germ cell function. *PLoS One.* 2008;3(2):e1571.
32. Bui HT, Van Thuan N, Kishigami S et al. Regulation of chromatin and chromosome morphology by histone H3 modifications in pig oocytes. *Reproduction.* 2007;133(2):371–82.
33. Tachibana M, Nozaki M, Takeda N, Shinkai Y. Functional dynamics of H3K9 methylation during meiotic prophase progression. *EMBO J.* 2007;26(14):3346–59.
34. Yoon J, Lee KS, Park JS, Yu K, Paik SG, Kang YK. dSETDB1 and SU (VAR)3-9 sequentially function during germline-stem cell differentiation in. *Drosophila melanogaster PLoS One.* 2008;3(5):e2234.
35. Aranda S, Mas G, Di Croce L. Regulation of gene transcription by polycomb proteins. *Sci Adv [Internet].* 2015;1(11):e1500737–e1500737. Available from: http://advances.sciencemag.org/cgi/doi/10.1126/sciadv.1500737
36. Scheuermann JC, De Ayala Alonso AG et al. Histone H2A deubiquitinase activity of the polycomb repressive complex PR-DUB. *Nature.* 2010;465(7295):243–7.
37. Stewart KR, Veselovska L, Kim J et al. Dynamic changes in histone modifications precede *de novo* DNA methylation in oocytes. *Genes Dev.* 2015;29(23):2449–62.
38. Edwards CA, Ferguson-Smith AC. Mechanisms regulating imprinted genes in clusters. *Curr Opin Cell Biol.* 2007;19:281–9.
39. Santos F, Peters AH, Otte AP, Reik W, Dean W. Dynamic chromatin modifications characterise the first cell cycle in mouse embryos. *Dev Biol.* 2005;280(1):225–36.
40. Eid A, Rodriguez-Terrones D, Burton A, Torres-Padilla ME. SUV4-20 activity in the preimplantation mouse embryo controls timely replication. *Genes Dev.* 2016;30(22):2513–26.
41. Zhou N, Cao Z, Wu R et al. Dynamic changes of histone H3 lysine 27 acetylation in pre implantational pig embryos derived from somatic cell nuclear transfer. *Anim Reprod Sci.* 2014;148(3–4):153–63.
42. Liu X, Wang C, Liu W et al. Distinct features of H3K4me3 and H3K27me3 chromatin domains in pre implantation embryos. *Nature.* 2016;537(7621):558–62.
43. Tachibana M, Sugimoto K, Nozaki M et al. G9a histone methyltransferase plays a dominant role in euchromatic histone H3 lysine 9 methylation and is essential for early embryogenesis. *Genes Dev.* 2002;16(14):1779–91.
44. Yamaguchi T, Cubizolles F, Zhang Y et al. Histone deacetylases 1 and 2 act in concert to promote the G1-to-S progression. *Genes Dev.* 2010;24(5):455–69.
45. Kawamura Y, Uchijima Y, Horike N et al. Sirt3 protects *in vitro*-fertilized mouse preimplantation embryos against oxidative stress-induced p53-mediated developmental arrest. *J Clin Invest.* 2010;120(8):2817–28.
46. Tahmasbpour E, Balasubramanian D, Agarwal A. A multi-faceted approach to understanding male infertility: Gene mutations, molecular defects and assisted reproductive techniques (ART). *J Assist Reprod Genet.* 2014;31:1115–37.
47. El Hajj N, Haaf T. Epigenetic disturbances in *in vitro* cultured gametes and embryos: Implications for human assisted reproduction. *Fertil Steril.* 2013;99:632–41.
48. Kohda T. Effects of embryonic manipulation and epigenetics. *J Hum Genet.* 2013;58:416–20.
49. Eroglu A, Layman LC. Role of ART in imprinting disorders. *Semin Reprod Med.* 2012;30(2):92–104.
50. Wang N, Le F, Zhan Q-T et al. Effects of *in vitro* maturation on histone acetylation in metaphase II oocytes and early cleavage embryos. *Obstet Gynecol Int [Internet].* 2010;2010:1–9. Available from: http://www.hindawi.com/journals/ogi/2010/989278/

51. Whitworth KM, Prather RS. Somatic cell nuclear transfer efficiency: How can it be improved through nuclear remodeling and reprogramming? *Mol Reprod Dev.* 2010;77:1001–15.

52. Iager AE, Ragina NP, Ross PJ et al. Trichostatin A improves histone acetylation in bovine somatic cell nuclear transfer early embryos. *Cloning Stem Cells [Internet].* 2008;10(3):371–9. Available from: http://www.ncbi.nlm.nih.gov/pubmed/18419249

53. Yan LY, Yan J, Qiao J, Zhao PL, Liu P. Effects of oocyte vitrification on histone modifications. *Reprod Fertil Dev.* 2010;22(6):920–5.

54. Wu FR, Liu Y, Shang MB et al. Differences in H3K4 trimethylation in *in vivo* and *in vitro* fertilization mouse preimplantation embryos. *Genet Mol Res.* 2012;11(2):1099–108.

55. Sutovsky P, Aarabi M, Miranda-Vizuete A, Oko R. Negative biomarker based male fertility evaluation: Sperm phenotypes associated with molecular-level anomalies. *Asian J Androl.* 2015;17(4):554–60. doi: 10.4103/1008-682X.153847.

56. Ge ZJ, Schatten H, Zhang CL, Sun QY. Oocyte ageing and epigenetics. *Reproduction.* 2015;149:R103–14.

CHAPTER 3

Epigenetic Reprogramming in Early Embryo Development

Sebastian Canovas and Pilar Coy

CONTENTS

3.1 INTRODUCTION

Early embryo development is usually understood as the stage between fertilization and blastocyst implantation, and the places where it physically befalls in mammals involve the uterine tube (oviduct, fallopian tube) and the uterus itself. Under the biological point of view, what happens during the early embryo development is that two highly specialized cells, the spermatozoon and the oocyte, fuse to later originate a number of "undifferentiated" or "non-specialized" cells, the 2, 4, 8, or successive multiples of blastomeres in the early embryos. Under the DNA methylation context, what happens is that two methylated genomes (the ones from the spermatozoon and the oocyte) fuse to originate one common genome that is progressively less methylated, as the blastomere divisions follow one another (1–3). In other words, and combining the biological and DNA methylation views, during early embryo development the cell type-specific epigenetic program disappears temporarily to, shortly after, begin to be re-written differentially according with the cell type.

In theory, this massive demethylation of the DNA has some exceptions: The imprinted genes and some active retrotransposons, which escape the process and maintain their DNA methylation marks through embryo divisions. In addition, not only DNA but also other epigenetic marks as histone modifications undergo drastic changes during this period in the life cycle. Through the following headings, four major questions will try to be answered: First, how and when does the DNA demethylation process of the paternal and maternal genomes (from gametes to blastocyst stager) occur? Second, why is this demethylation necessary and what is its evolutionary impact? Third, why and how do the imprinted genes and active retrotransposons escape this event and what are the consequences of such methylation maintenance? And finally, what happens with histone epigenetic marks and how do they correlate with the DNA methylation changes?

3.2 HOW AND WHEN ARE THE PATERNAL AND MATERNAL GENOMES DEMETHYLATED DURING THE PREIMPLANTATION PERIOD?

The first issue to clarify, before knowing "how" or "when," is "what" DNA demethylation means in the current context. In general, demethylation implies the loss of 5-methyl-cytosines (5mC) present in the DNA sequence of gametes which can be re-converted into cytosines (C) or thymines (T) as explained in previous chapters. These 5mC appear usually in a symmetrical pattern, that is, both strands at the cytosine-guanine dinucleotides (CpG) carry the cytosine modification. Usually, CpGs appear in clusters throughout the genome forming the so-called "CpG islands" (CpGi), most frequently located in the promoter region and first exon of genes (4). Demethylation then, occurs when the methyl group of the C is lost and this loss can be produced either by the action of specific enzymes (active demethylation) or simply by the division of the cell, when DNA replication occurs without the subsequent establishment of methylations at the new C of the recently formed strand (passive demethylation, Figure 3.1).

DNA methylation marks affect transcription and readout of the DNA. In general, the presence of 5mC in specific genome features (mainly CpGi at the promoters) may decide if the downstream sequence will be or not be transcribed, determining then the fate of the cell containing that genome. Overall, the consequence of the loss of 5mC along a genome is the lack of marks indicating which parts of that genome must not be transcribed (Figure 3.2). This means that, in adult tissues, the cells show different methylation patterns that

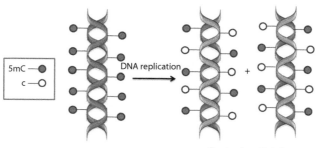

FIGURE 3.1 Schematic representation of the passive DNA demethylation process during DNA replication. In absence of DNA methyltransferase activity, the 5mC positions are substituted in the new formed strand by C, producing a dilution effect on the balance of DNA methylation.

influence which genes are expressed or repressed and, consequently, which types of cells that tissue contains and which function develops.

The knowing of the specific dynamics of C methylation during the early development period is crucial to understand the future consequences that each specific alteration in the reprogramming of the genome can have. The initial studies, showing a loss of methylation in the male and female genomes as the zygote progressed in its development and started to cleave, made global measurements by means of non-quantitative or semi-quantitative techniques, including DNA electrophoresis and Southern blot (1) or immunofluorescence (3,5). Also, targeted analysis at individual *loci* using bisulfite sequencing was depicted (6). From the initial studies it was established that, in general, the maternal genome was passively demethylated during replication (Figure 3.1) and the paternal genome was actively demethylated by the action of the ten-eleven-translocation (TET) enzymes although, as it will

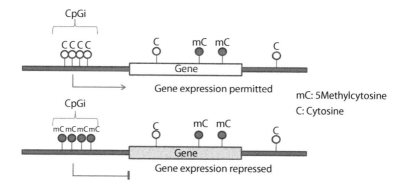

FIGURE 3.2 Theoretical effect, for a downstream gene, of methylation at cytosines located in a CpG island (CpGi) at the gene promoter.

be further discussed, this concept has been re-interpreted. These TET enzymes oxidize 5mC to 5-hydroximethylcytosine (5hmC) and later to other forms such as 5-formylcytosine (5fC) and 5-carboxylcytosine (5caC). The importance of this oxidization is that the effect produced by the 5mC on the DNA (i.e., deciding the repression of transcription at a specific sequence) is modified when 5hmC or other C forms occupies those loci and so the epigenetic message is altered. In theory, 5hmC is only poorly recognised by DNA-methyl transferase enzymes (DNMT) and its presence can lead to passive demethylation by preventing maintenance methylation after replication (reviewed by Reference 7). The TET family consists of at least three members (TET1, TET2, and TET3). During early embryo development, TET3 seems to play a prominent role, since its expression is high in oocytes and decreases rapidly as the blastocyst appears. In contrast, TET1 and TET2 are highly expressed in the inner cell mass (ICM) of the blastocyst and later, TET1 begins to be downregulated but TET2 and TET3 either remain constant or are upregulated as cell differentiation progresses (8). While TET enzymes are responsible for hydroxymethylation and subsequent demethylation by lack of maintenance methylation after replication, DNMT enzymes, as above mentioned, are responsible for DNA methylation and work in collaboration with a family of proteins that contain conserved methyl-CpG binding domains (MBDs) and recognize sites of DNA methylation (9). Briefly, DNMT1 is considered responsible for maintaining the methylation pattern in a new DNA strand after replication (10) while DNMT3A and DNMT3B usually perform *de novo* DNA methylation at previously unmethylated CpGs. However, it was shown that all the three enzymes are capable of both activities with different efficiency (11). Also, there are other factors modulating DNMT activities such as a nuclear protein of 95 kDa (NP95, also known as UHRF1) and DNMT3L. While DNMT3L stimulates DNMT3A and DNMT3B activity (12), maternal UHRF1 is essential for maintaining CG methylation at the imprinting control regions (13) (see Reference 7 for review).

Focusing on the DNA demethylation process during early embryo development, there has been a number of studies describing it during pronuclear development, short after fertilization (2,14–17). However, there are scarce reports showing, on a quantitative, genome-wide scale, the whole reprogramming process from gametes to blastocyst in mammals, and all of them have been performed on biological samples coming from human (18,19), mouse (20), or monkey (21). From this information, some common patterns in all these species could be now accepted, and are represented in Figure 3.3. In addition, a detailed description of what is known and could be different between species at every specific stage is summarized in the following sections.

DNA Methylation Dynamics from Gametes to Zygote and 2-Cell Stage

The first and deep global drop in the 5mC levels (DNA demethylation) can be observed a few hours after fertilization and it is especially evident in the male genome (Figure 3.3). For

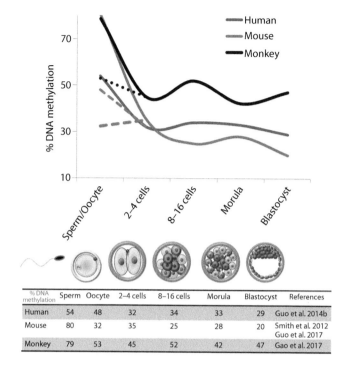

% DNA methylation	Sperm	Oocyte	2–4 cells	8–16 cells	Morula	Blastocyst	References
Human	54	48	32	34	33	29	Guo et al. 2014b
Mouse	80	32	35	25	28	20	Smith et al. 2012 Guo et al. 2017
Monkey	79	53	45	52	42	47	Gao et al. 2017

FIGURE 3.3 Global DNA methylation levels at different stages during preimplantational embryo development in human, mouse, and monkey species. Dashed lines start at the global methylation level of the oocyte while the continuous lines start at the spermatozoa methylation level. Drops in global DNA methylation from gametes to 2–4-cell stage are close: Mouse spermatozoa show 80% of global methylation and mouse oocyte 32% (figurative arithmetic mean value for both gametes being 56%) with methylation dropping down to 35% at 2-cell stage, that is, a global 21% decrease (20,22); human spermatozoa and oocyte show less differences between them (54% vs. 48%; arithmetic mean 51%), with methylation at 2-cell stage dropping to 32%, meaning a global 19% decrease (18); finally, monkey spermatozoa showed 79% of global methylation and oocyte gave a value of 53% (arithmetic mean 65%), being at 2-cell stage 45%, which again represents a global 20% decrease (21). The importance of such absolute values could be irrelevant because differences in the procedures and samples can affect these figures but the similarity in the decrease can be considered of around the same magnitude in the three species.

this reason, initial studies in mouse suggested that such paternal demethylation process was active and mediated by TET enzymes (2). Similarly, it was considered that maternal genome demethylation was probably due to a replication-dependent dilution process (passive demethylation) and, for this reason demethylation appeared later, as the cell divisions progressed. In this same species (mouse), it was later observed, by immunostaining, that 5hmC, 5fC, and 5caC appeared in the male pronucleus as 5mC was disappearing, and that the two last forms (5fC and 5caC) remained in the zygote showing passive dilution by replication instead of being actively removed, suggesting a role in the epigenetic message for these forms (14).

However, studies in isolated male and female pronuclei, using reduced representation bisulfite sequencing (RRBS) to evaluate genome-wide DNA methylation, and using aphidicolin to inhibit DNA replication, showed a marked reduction in methylated cytosines in both male and female genomes in absence of cell division (16,17), as previously suggested (15). These data demonstrated active removal of methylation mediated by TET3 in both parental genomes, particularly at certain *loci*, although to a lesser extent in the maternal than in the paternal DNA. Despite this, the authors concluded that DNA replication is the major contributor to paternal and maternal DNA demethylation as the zygote starts to divide and that TET3 facilitates DNA demethylation by coupling with DNA replication. Although all these experiments were performed in mice, a recent study in monkey has also shown that that both paternal and maternal genomes undergo active DNA demethylation (21).

DNA Methylation Dynamics from 2- to 8-Cell Stage

According to the available information, the global methylation percentage from the 2-cell stage to the 8-cell stage continues slightly falling in the mouse, while the values are either similar in human (18) or higher in monkey (21) as development progresses through this temporal window (Figure 3.3), raising the question of whether active and passive demethylation are slowing down (in the human case), or whether active *de novo* methylation (by DNMT3A/DNMT3B) or remethylation (by DNMT1) processes are growing (in the monkey case). For passive demethylation, it is unlikely to stop under a period of continuous cell divisions unless DNMT1 activity increases. As the number of *DNMT1* transcripts from maternal origin in the cytoplasm cannot increase at this stage, the possible answer should be searched in the fact that DNMT1 from the embryo begins to be highly expressed. In the mouse, DNMT1 is excluded from nuclei of cleavage embryos (22) and, according to Hirasawa et al. (23), "the vast majority of the DNMT1 proteins present in preimplantation embryos are of maternal origin" so that, at least in this species, an increase in DNMT1 activity is not plausible and this option would not be valid to explain, in a global methylation context, that remethylation dominated over demethylation at this time in the mouse species, as indeed is not hapening. In the monkey, since DNMT1 does not seem to be more highly expressed at the 8-cell stage than at the 2-cell stage or morula (21), the action of this enzyme cannot be the answer for the question about the observed remethylation wave. Also, DNMT3a, or DNMT3a1, does not change drastically from the oocyte to the morula (Figure 3.4), and DNMT3a2 and DNMT3b almost disappear at the 8-cell and morula stages, discarding the option that an increase in the *de novo* methylation can explain this observation. Having said that, the last chance to explain the monkey data could be a downregulation in oxidative

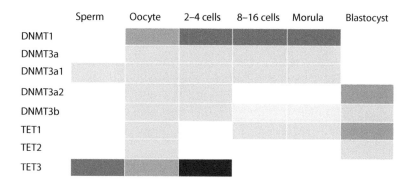

FIGURE 3.4 Relative expression levels of the DNMT and TET protein families through the early embryo development. The more intense the blue color, the higher expression of a particular protein (8,18,25,26).

demethylation by TETs. According to Gao et al. (21), at the 8-cell stage TET3 expression is almost zero, and TET1 and TET2 are just beginning to be expressed which could entail a low oxidative demethylation activity around an 8–16-cell stage, with a subsequent increase at the morula stage. However, a similar pattern of TET´s expression also exists in the mouse (24), where the remethylation wave observed in the monkey at this stage is not present, so that this explanation is neither the answer to the question. Also, the same changes have been shown in the pig, where TET3 enzymes showed high expression at the zygote and 2-cell stage but lower expression at the 4-cell stage, and TET1 increased at the morula and bastocyst stages (25). The whole methylation landscape at high resolution, high coverage, in this latter species during early development is not yet available, so that, even though the TET enzymes pattern at this period seems evolutionary conserved, it is unknown if the remethylation wave observed in monkey is shared by other species. Since the authors did not propose a mechanism to explain their observation but a recent study has also shown the occurrence of remethylation activity in the mouse zygote (26), it could be a hypothesis to explore the relationship between the time of zygote genome activation (ZGA) in each species and the observation of remethylation phenomena. In fact, from Gao et al.'s study (21) the main conclusion is that DNA methylation dynamics at preimplantation embryos is not unidirectional and that both DNA demethylation and *de novo* methylation take place simultaneously, affecting different *loci*. This suggests that remethylation can be playing a role in the fine-tune regulation of the gene expression at this stage or, as it was already suggested for demethylation (27), can influence transcriptional activation.

As it is already known, the embryo is transcriptionally quiescent at the initial stages, and only the maternal proteins and RNAs in the zygote cytoplasm lead the development. Later on, during the maternal-to-zygotic transition, the control is taken by the activated nuclear genome of the zygote itself, and this is also a phenomenon displayed on sequential waves (28), occurring in the major ZGA wave in humans at the 4–8-cell stage (29) and at the 2-cell stage in the mouse (28), having been associated to DNA demethylation (25,27). Since ZGA has similar time frames in the monkey than in humans (30,31), could it then be a plausible idea that the remethylation waves, observed at the zygote stage in the mouse (26) and at the 8-cell stage in the monkey (21) were, in some way, also connected with the ZGA waves and could play a role in its regulation, for instance, modifying the chromatin structure or recruiting other transcriptional machinery.

DNA Methylation Dynamics from 8- to 16-Cell Stage to Morula

After the 8–16-cell stage and onto the morula stage, demethylation again dominates over remethylation in monkey, falling down the global percentage (53%–42%), but seeming to keep approximately steady in human (34%–33%) and mouse (28%–30%) (Figure 3.3). At this time, the ZGA is already established in all the three species and the first cell fate lineage begins to be drawn. Also, TET3 almost disappear and TET1 and TET2 are close to assume their roles for the oxidative demethylation (Figure 3.3), together with replication dependent passive demethylation, although the possibility of some other yet unknown factors playing a role in this process cannot be discarded. DNMT1, however, keeps highly expressed at this time frame (21) guaranteeing methylation maintenance as the divisions progresses, at least at certain *loci*, as it will be later explained.

DNA Methylation Dynamics from the Morula to the Blastocyst Stage

Finally, at the blastocyst stage, the global DNA methylation level reaches their lowest values in the human (29%) and mouse (19%–21%) species although in the monkey it is slightly higher than in morula (42% vs. 47%). It is important to point out that the mentioned values have been obtained from the ICM and not from the whole blastocyst although, from the available data in mouse, with similar values in both the ICM and the trophectoderm (21% and 19%, respectively) (32), and from our data reported in other species such as the cow (22% vs. 21% for ICM and TE [trophectoderm], respectively) (33), or even the pig, which shows the lowest values of global DNA methylation reported in the whole blastocyst (15%) (34), it is not expected a high variation between both cell lineages in the human data, remaining unknown if the case would be the same in the monkey.

3.3 WHY IS THIS DEMETHYLATION NECESSARY? WHAT IS ITS EVOLUTIONARY IMPACT?

Once explained how demethylation occurs in the preimplantation embryo (although, from the data above detailed, it is a more drastic event for the male genome than for the female one), the first answer to the question of why demethylation is necessary comes up from the need of the embryo to be made up of totipotent cells before initiating the differentiation process. The Nature has devised a smart mechanism to de-program the genome of two highly specialized cells and transform them in a "blank check" (with exceptions that will be further discussed), which is blanker as the number of cells increases from the zygote to the blastocyst, when the cell lineages start again to be drawn.

From an evolutionary point of view, DNA methylation and other epigenetic marks (such as histone methylation, histone acetylation and de-acetylation) represent a more rapid response to environmental changes than evolution via genetic mutation, the way followed by natural selection (35). Not in vain, epigenetics is defined "as heritable but potentially reversible changes in gene expression caused by mechanisms other than changes in the underlying DNA sequence" (36). In fact, changes in gene expression derived from epigenetic modifications can occur in one organism during embryonic or fetal development, or during adulthood, and can persist through generations, as the classical examples used to explain the concept of Epigenetics usually refers: The alterations found as a consequence of the Dutch Famine of 1944–1945, explained by the so-called Developmental Origins of Health and Disease (DOHaD) hypothesis (37).

However, despite there are many studies showing direct correlations between alterations in the conditions surrounding the preimplantation embryos in the oviduct, and overall the fetus in the uterus, and their post-birth or adulthood health, the opposite has been far less investigated: What are the ideal conditions regarding nutrients availability, temperature, blood flow, oxygen or CO_2 levels, to let the embryo develops in absence of stress? In other words, what are the conditions that evolution would "naturally select" to avoid mistakes in the epigenetic context and produce the best adapted individuals? Some examples can help to clarify this idea. For instance, it seems now clear that by changing the availability of methyl donors in the diet it is possible to modify the kinetics of DNA and histone methylation, thereby modulating the epigenetic landscape (35). The best known example is that of the agouti gene in mouse, whose expression is controlled by the methylation at the 5′ long terminal repeat (LTR) of the Intracisternal A-particles (IAPs) retrotransposon (38). In this mouse, it was demonstrated that maternal dietary methyl supplements increased the level of DNA methylation in the agouti LTR and changed the phenotype of offspring, producing the favorable one (healthier and of longest life). Some other examples related with the benefits of methyl donors in the diet, such as choline, folic acid, vitamin B_1, betaine, and methionine can be found in the literature and this concept has been referred as "epigenetic rescue by diet" (35). These compounds, supplemented during gestation, can mitigate the effects of maternal obesity on offspring (39); also, when administered during post-natal development, can help to produce carcass of greater value as it was shown in cattle (40); or, as it was shown for the mammary tumours in rats supplemented with methyl donors during puberty, they can help reduce the cancer risk (41). Other factors in the environment that can affect the epigenetic reprogramming in the preimplantation embryo include the temperature, the ROS and O_2 levels, directly related with TET activity, or the use of assisted reproductive technologies, which fairly influence multiple conditions during the first week of development (42–44).

What could be the impact of these findings from the evolutionary point of view? If we knew the precise epigenetic marks needed to adapt to e environmental conditions during development or to reduce cancer, improve health or increase life expectancy, we would have a powerful tool to influence evolution and to speed up selection of specific traits since those favorable epigenetic marks could be transmitted to the offspring. On the other way around, this same knowledge could help to reverse or delete aberrant epigenetic marks emerged as a consequence of any kind of stress in one organism and to avoid the problem was inherited by the next generation (7). Some interesting studies showing the critical role played by DNA methylation in evolution of duplicate genes (45) or explaining how to design strategies capable of predicting the relationships among DNA methylation, the early environment of an organism, and its phenotype in a future environment (46) also support this thesis.

3.4 WHY AND HOW THE IMPRINTED GENES AND ACTIVE RETROTRANSPOSON ARE NOT DEMETHYLATED

As already discussed in previous chapters, genomic imprinting is a phenomenon by which only one copy of a gene (either paternal or maternal) is expressed, remaining silent the other copy (36). Thus, genomic imprinting represents a greater genomic risk for mammals because a genetic or epigenetic mutation in one allele can result in the absence of crucial gene products and lead to a number of imprinting disorders causing different syndromes (47,48).

As explained in previous chapters, most of the imprinting genes are clustered into 16 genomic regions and those clusters contain not only paternal and maternal protein-coding RNAs but also a non-coding RNA (ncRNA) and an imprint control region (ICR), that exhibits parental allele-specific DNA methylation and post-translational histone modifications (36,49). Depending upon the gene, methylation of the ICR may silence the gene by blocking the binding of transcription factors or enhancers, or activate the gene by blocking the binding of insulators, which repress transcription (50). Thus, in contrast to what it has been explained in this chapter as a general rule, the study of imprinting genes led to discover that "one biological role of DNA methylation is to allow expression of genes normally repressed by default" (36).

Imprinting occurs with less than 2% of genes, which in mammals represents almost two hundred genes, and many of these genes are essential for proper embryo, fetal, and placental function and development, as well as for X chromosome inactivation (47,51,52). The loss of imprinting in the preimplantational embryo would result in a not viable product due to the over expression of these specific genes during development (53). For this reason, the global DNA demethylation wave occurring at this stage should not affect these specific features (Figure 3.5); also, other epigenetic marks at the imprinted genes inherited from the gametes into the zygote must be maintained throughout embryonic development. But, how can this be achieved?

To let imprints escape genome-wide reprogramming occurring after fertilization, active demethylation on the paternally methylated alleles must be prevented but, as the embryo development progresses, it is also crucial that these regions survive the subsequent

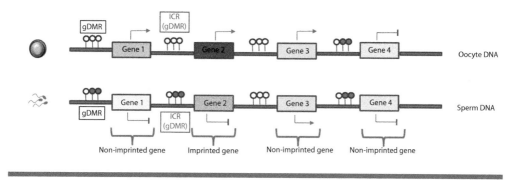

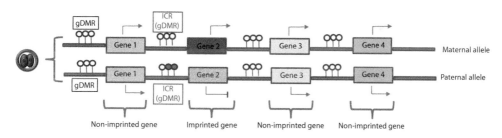

FIGURE 3.5   Simplified representation for the putative effect of the first DNA demethylation wave post-fertilization on different genes. Four genes in the oocyte and spermatozoon (top) and in the 2-cell stage embryo (bottom) DNA are depicted. The gamete differentially methylated region–gDMR (black) controls the expression of Gene 1 (yellow), which is silenced in the male gamete but not in the oocyte. After fertilization and first cleavage, demethylation at the gDMR results in the expression of both alleles. For the paternally imprinted Gene 2 (pink), the gDMR (red) functions as an imprinting control region (ICR), which escapes the demethylation wave thus maintaining the paternal allele silenced at the 2-cell stage embryo. Gene 3 (blue) is not differentially methylated between the oocyte and the spermatozoon and its expression is not repressed by DNA methylation so that is not affected by the demethylation wave after fertilization. Gene 4 (green) is repressed in the gametes but, after demethylation becomes "released" in both alleles of the 2-cell stage embryo, contributing to totipotency of the blastomeres.

wave of *de novo* methylation (54), one of which occurs, at least in the monkey example referred at the beginning of this chapter, as soon as at the 8–16-cell stage (21). Also, as the division frequency increases, the DNA methylation and other epigenetic modifications must be copied on the newly replicated DNA. To accomplish these complex tasks, different mechanisms are necessary.

The first and essential mechanism by which the imprints are maintained is by the action of the oocyte-specific isoform of DNMT1, called DNMT1o, that maintains the imprints at one single cell cycle in preimplantation development (22). Also, the somatic form of DNMT1, expressed in the zygote, DNMT1s, maintains the methylation pattern at imprinting regions until the morula stage (55) with the only exception of Rasgrf1 differentially methylated region (DMR), which requires zygotic Dnmt3b for the imprint maintenance (23,56). However, it is still unknown how DNMT1o or DNMT1a can find the gamete differentially methylated regions (gDMRs) in the genome (57) or specific imprinting control regions (ICRs) and protect them from demethylation. In mouse some specific paternal imprinted loci are protected from the demehtylation through TET3 hydroxilation, by the binding of PGC7 to H3K9me2 at these specific foci (58).

A second protective mechanism against DNA demethylation is mediated by DNA-binding factors that can specifically recognize ICRs and avoid demethylation (47). One of these factors is MBD3, which binds indirectly to methylated cytosine as part of a complex, and maintains methylation silencing the paternally imprinted allele H19 (59). Another protein that has been shown to contribute the imprint maintenance is ZFP57, a maternal transcription factor presents in early embryos. Lack of both maternal and zygotic ZFP57 results in embryonic lethality and complete loss of methylation at the Snrpn, Peg1, Peg3, Peg5, and Dlk1 DMRs (60). Other proteins with significant roles in this function are PGC7 (or STELLA) whose lack produce a global loss of DNA methylation on the maternal pronucleus of the zygote (61) and RBBP1/ARID4A and RBBP1L1/ARID4B, which are also involved in maintenance of imprinting at the Snprn locus(62). In addition, it has been reported in mouse maternal H3K27me3 as a DNA methylation-independent imprinting mechanism. It shows a radical difference to DNA methylation-dependent imprinting, because it is maintained in preimplantation embryos but is diluted in ICM and almost undetectable in the epiblast of E6.5 embryos, although in some gene it stays longer (E9.5) in placenta (63).

Despite the mentioned factors, our knowledge of the epigenetic mechanisms maintaining and protecting imprints during early embryo development is still incomplete, and it is likely that new factors will be identified in the following years. In addition, apart from imprinting genes, there is another genome feature escaping DNA demethylation during this period, namely certain active pieces of mobile DNA known as transposable elements (TEs). TEs, also named "the jumping genes," are DNA sequences discovered in the 50 s in maize (64) and these sequences can move from one location to another in the genome. In humans, TEs comprise an astonishing 50% of our genome (65,66).

In eukaryotes, two main types of TEs have been described, retrotransposons and DNA transposons. DNA transposons or class II TEs move by a simple "cut and paste" mechanism: A DNA transposon sequence is removed from one genomic location and inserted in a new genomic site, using a specialized protein termed transposase (67). Its proportion in the human and mouse genome is lower than 5%, and no active DNA-transposons are present in these genomes at present. On the other hand, retrotransposons, or class I TEs, move by a "copy and paste" mechanism of mobilization that requires reverse transcription of an intermediate TEs RNA. In the human and mouse, more than 95% of TEs belong to this class (66) and represent more than 35% of the genome (68).

Notably, active retrotransposons are currently mobilizing in the human and mouse genome (69). Retrotransposons are also divided in two types, those containing long-terminal repeats (LTRs) on both ends, known as LTR retrotransposons or endogenous retroviruses (ERVs), and those lacking LTRs, non-LTR retrotransposons. Although in mouse both LTR and non-LTR retrotransposons continue to generate interindividual genomic variability, in humans only retrotransposons from the non-LTR retrotransposon class are currently active. Within non-LTR retrotransposons, two main types of elements can be described: The SINE family (short interspersed elements) and the LINE family (long interspersed elements). SINEs are short and non-coding sequences, while LINEs are coding sequences that generate protein products responsible for the mobilization of both LINEs and SINEs. Within LINEs, the class 1 of these elements (LINE-1s) is the evolutionary younger family of elements that continue to generate variability in our genome. From a copy number perspective, SINE elements such as Alu have accumulated more than a million copies over human evolution, while LINE-1s have generated a substantial half million copies over evolution. In sum, both LINE-1s and SINEs make up an estimated 15%–17% of the human genome due to its length (70,71).

As active pieces of mobile DNA, the activity of LINE-1 and SINE, moving through the genome, can cause mutations when they are inserted inside a gene, being involved in different diseases such as hemophilia (72) or colon cancer (73), but also contributing genetic diversity (68). In the mouse, an incidence of 1 or more LINE-1 insertions per every eight births has been recently reported (74).

During preimplantation development, most retrotransposons are demethylated following the general pattern of the rest of the genome. That makes them pass from the "silent" to the "active" stage and this activity has been associated with some of the earliest transcriptional events during zygotic genome activation and has also been considered a general requirement for progression through cleavage (75,76). Recently, by manipulation of the expression of young LINE-1 members in mouse, a study suggested that LINE-1 transcription during early embryo development affects chromatin condensation and it could impact developmental rates. In fact, premature silencing of LINE-1 decreases chromatin decondensation, whereas prolonged LINE-1 activation interferes gradual recondensation that is necessary for normal developmental progression and decreases developmental rates (77).

Indeed, in the mouse genome the discovery that L1Md-A elements within the LINE-1 family and the Class II IAPs within the LTR retrotransposons hold higher methylation levels upon fertilization and throughout cleavage (20,78) opened the question of whether these particular elements may play an specific role that make them necessary to remain silent in this period. As above explained, IAP methylation contribute to epigenetic inheritance of the favorable phenotype of the agouti gene in mouse, and also to variability between individuals and to avoid other mutations (78). As far as for LINE-1 is concerned, it was shown in human embryos that young LINE-1 elements are more resistant to demethylation than their older counterparts probably to maintain stronger repression of their transcription and activity by DNA methylation (18). However, it remains to be investigated how this methylation maintenance occurs and what its real function is during development. In summary, TEs are a source of genetic diversity and an important part of evolution but, at the same time, the genome must partially inhibit their activity to keep the balance in the gene regulation of the organism (79).

3.5 WHAT HAPPENS WITH HISTONE EPIGENETIC MARKS AND HOW DO THEY CORRELATE WITH THE DNA METHYLATION CHANGES?

Histones are proteins that associate with DNA to package chromatin into nucleosomes which allows DNA condensation but also restricts access of regulatory factors to the DNA strand, affecting transcription. Histone tails are exposed on the nucleosome surface and they can be modified by addition of different molecules (acetylation, methylation, but also ubiquitination, SUMOylation, and phosphorylation) which alters the chromatin structure and increase or reduce its accessibility, according with the specific residue and/or the number of molecules that are added to histone amino acids. Histone tails modifications can correlate with different biological effects including DNA repression or activation, and configure a complex marking system called "histone code" (80,81). For example, histone acetylation affects chromatin structure (by decreasing interaction between positive charges on the histones and the negatively charged DNA) and facilitates the access of transcription factors to DNA. However, according with position and the number of methyl groups that are added to histone tails, it can correlate with either silencing (H3K9me3 and H3K27me3) or with activation (H3K4me3, H3K36me3) of DNA. But also histones modifications are connected to DNA methylation machinery or even protection of DNA from demethylation (82).

Drastic changes of the histone tail modifications during the preimplantational period have been reported and detailed information is available in recent reviews by different authors including ourselves (7,83–85). Briefly, histone remodeling starts, just after sperm-egg fusion, with the replacement of protamines by oocyte-derived histones in the sperm, which entails an epigenetic asymmetry between pronucleus, with an initial predominance of acetylated and unmethylated histones in the spermatozoa. Overall, modifications associated with gene repression (H3K27me3, H3K9me2/me3) are deleted and there is an increase of activation marks (H3K4me3), concomitant with pluripotency acquisition. Later, inhibitory and other histone marks are reacquired at the initial steps of differentiation in the late blastocyst, showing asymmetrical distribution between ICM and TE although these differences are not directly correlated with gene transcription (86).

However, information about genome-wide histone tail modifications is scarce, in part due to the limitations to obtain the size of the sample that requires this technique ($\sim$10,000 cells). During the last 2–3 years, different approaches have used low-input systems coupled with chromatin immunoprecipitation sequencing (ChIP-Seq) and provided first panoramic views of the landscape of different histone marks during early embryo stages (87). This genome-wide information is helpful to clarify connections between DNA methylation and histone tail modifications. There are some evidences that suggest that histone tail marks can modulate accessibility of the readers of DNA methylation to chromatin but these two layers of epigenetic marks are interconnected through different pathways (Figure 3.6).

H3K9 methylation is one example of interconnection between histone marks and DNA methylation maintenance machinery, but not the unique. They play key roles in the control of DNA methylation by mediate, through UHRF1, the target of DNMT1 for DNA methylation (88). UHRF1, an essential cofactor of DNMT1, contains two domains (TUDOR and PHD) that participate in the binding of UHRF1 to methylated-H3K9 which favors DNMT1 targeting for the maintenance of DNA methylation (88–91). H3K27me3, another repressive mark, is catalyzed by the Polycomb Repressive Complex 2 (PRC2), and it is deleted during early development and reacquired at differentiation in the blastocyst. It is present in many key developmental genes and regulators of pluripotency and is under a tightly regulation for successful embryo development (92,93). However, its relationship with DNA methylation remains poorly characterized, even it is known that H3K27me3 and DNA methylation tend to be mutually exclusive in CpGi (94). The general proposed mechanism implies that the preexisting absence of DNA methylation is required, but not sufficient, for H3K27 methylation and the sequence (mainly CpG density) and transcriptional activation impose constraints on PCR2 activity. Exclusion of DNMTs by PRC2 has been linked to TET1 to avoid DNA methylation from H3K27me3 enriched-CpG island in embryonic stem cells (95).

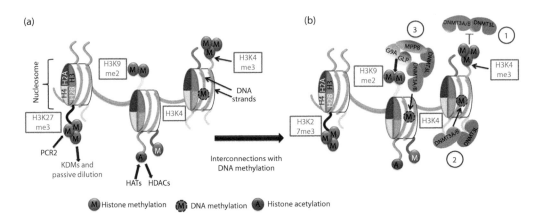

FIGURE 3.6 (a) Main repressive (H3K27me3, H3K9me3) and active (H3K4me2/3) histone modifications during embryo development and relevant enzymes which participate in the addition or removal of these modifications. HATs: Histone acetyltransferases; HDACs: Histone deacetylases; KDMs: Lysine demethylases; PRC2 Polycomb repressive complex 2; Nucleosome consisting of DNA coiled around a octamer of histones (H2A, H2B, H3, and H4). (b) Examples of interconnections between histones modifications and DNA methylation. (1) H3K4me3 blocks interaction of DNMT3 enzymes with DNA and *de novo* DNA methylation is disabled in this loci. (2) When H3K4 is unmodified, DNMT3 domains interact with H3K4 and *de novo* DNA methylation activity by DNMT3A/B and DNMT3L is released.

Also, H3K4 methylation and *de novo* DNA methylation are interconnected. Active promoters are prevented from *de novo* methylation, between other mechanisms, through recruitment of H3K4 methyltransferases. The DNMT3 enzymes contain an ADD domain (ATRX– DNMT3–DNMT3L) that specifically require interacts with unmethylated H3K4, and this binding is blocked when H3K4 is methylated (96).

H3K9me2 is also interconnected with *de novo* DNA methylation and there is a high correlation between both epigenetic marks. G9A and G9L are the enzymes that add methyl groups at H3K9 and they influence *de novo* DNA methylation directly by recruitment of DNMT3A and DNMT3B (97,98). In addition, H3K9me2 also participate in the protection of DNA from demethylation. In mouse maternal genome and some specific paternal imprinted loci are protected from the demehtylation wave that takes place after fertilization, through TET3 hydroxilation, by the binding of PGC7 to H3K9me2 at these specific foci (58).

In conclusion, epigenetic remodeling is a complex and dynamic process that include DNA methylation, histone modifications and other epigenetic mechanisms. All together are regulated on a global scale but also tightly regulation at specific loci has been reported. Genome-wide analysis is helping to uncover the bases of these processes and this knowledge will help us to approach fertility studies and design new strategies, protocols, and treatments for infertility.

ACKNOWLEDGMENTS

The authors thank the funding received from the Regional Agency of Science (Fundacion Seneca), Murcia, Spain (Grant 20040/GERM/16).

REFERENCES

1. Monk M, Boubelik M, Lehnert S. Temporal and regional changes in DNA methylation in the embryonic, extraembryonic, and germ cell lineages during mouse embryo development. *Development*. 1987;99(3):371–82.
2. Oswald J, Engemann S, Lane N et al. Active demethylation of the paternal genome in the mouse zygote. *Curr Biol*. 2000;10(8):475–8.
3. Mayer W, Niveleau A, Walter J, Fundele R, Haaf T. Demethylation of the zygotic paternal genome. *Nature*. 2000;403(6769):501–2.
4. Larsen F, Gundersen G, Lopez R, Prydz H. CpG islands as gene markers in the human genome. *Genomics*. 1992;13(4):1095–107.
5. Barton SC, Arney KL, Shi W et al. Genome-wide methylation patterns in normal and uniparental early mouse embryos. *Hum Mol Genet*. 2001;10(26):2983–7.
6. Kim SH, Kang YK, Koo DB et al. Differential DNA methylation reprogramming of various repetitive sequences in mouse preimplantation embryos. *Biochem Biophys Res Commun*. 2004;324(1):58–63.
7. Ross PJ, Canovas S. Mechanisms of epigenetic remodelling during preimplantation development. *Reprod Fertil Dev*. 2016;28(1–2):25–40.
8. Rasmussen KD, Helin K. Role of TET enzymes in DNA methylation, development, and cancer. *Genes Dev*. 2016;30(7):733–50.
9. Law JA, Jacobsen SE. Establishing, maintaining, and modifying DNA methylation patterns in plants and animals. *Nat Rev Genet*. 2010;11(3):204–20.
10. Athanasiadou R, de Sousa D, Myant K, Merusi C, Stancheva I, Bird A. Targeting of *de novo* DNA methylation throughout the Oct-4 gene regulatory region in differentiating embryonic stem cells. *PLoS One*. 2010;5(4):e9937.
11. Arand J, Spieler D, Karius T et al. *In vivo* control of CpG and non-CpG DNA methylation by DNA methyltransferases. *PLoS Genet*. 2012;8(6):e1002750.
12. Bourc'his D, Xu GL, Lin CS, Bollman B, Bestor TH. Dnmt3L and the establishment of maternal genomic imprints. *Science*. 2001;294(5551):2536–9.
13. Maenohara S, Unoki M, Toh H et al. Role of UHRF1 in *de novo* DNA methylation in oocytes and maintenance methylation in preimplantation embryos. *PLoS Genet*. 2017;13(10):e1007042.
14. Inoue A, Shen L, Dai Q, He C, Zhang Y. Generation and replication-dependent dilution of 5fC and 5caC during mouse preimplantation development. *Cell Res*. 2011;21(12):1670–6.
15. Wang L, Zhang J, Duan J et al. Programming and inheritance of parental DNA methylomes in mammals. *Cell*. 2014;157(4):979–91.
16. Guo F, Li X, Liang D et al. Active and passive demethylation of male and female pronuclear DNA in the mammalian zygote. *Cell Stem Cell*. 2014;15(4):447–59.
17. Shen L, Inoue A, He J, Liu Y, Lu F, Zhang Y. Tet3 and DNA replication mediate demethylation of both the maternal and paternal genomes in mouse zygotes. *Cell Stem Cell*. 2014;15(4):459–71.
18. Guo H, Zhu P, Yan L et al. The DNA methylation landscape of human early embryos. *Nature*. 2014;511(7511):606–10.

19. Smith ZD, Chan MM, Humm KC et al. DNA methylation dynamics of the human preimplantation embryo. *Nature*. 2014;511(7511):611–5.

20. Smith ZD, Chan MM, Mikkelsen TS et al. A unique regulatory phase of DNA methylation in the early mammalian embryo. *Nature*. 2012;484(7394):339–44.

21. Gao F, Niu Y, Sun YE et al. De novo DNA methylation during monkey pre-implantation embryogenesis. *Cell Res*. 2017;27(4):526–39.

22. Howell CY, Bestor TH, Ding F et al. Genomic imprinting disrupted by a maternal effect mutation in the Dnmt1 gene. *Cell*. 2001;104(6):829–38.

23. Hirasawa R, Chiba H, Kaneda M et al. Maternal and zygotic Dnmt1 are necessary and sufficient for the maintenance of DNA methylation imprints during preimplantation development. *Genes Dev*. 2008;22(12):1607–16.

24. Iqbal K, Jin SG, Pfeifer GP, Szabó PE. Reprogramming of the paternal genome upon fertilization involves genome-wide oxidation of 5-methylcytosine. *Proc Natl Acad Sci USA*. 2011;108(9):3642–7.

25. Lee K, Hamm J, Whitworth K et al. Dynamics of TET family expression in porcine preimplantation embryos is related to zygotic genome activation and required for the maintenance of NANOG. *Dev Biol*. 2014;386(1):86–95.

26. Amouroux R, Nashun B, Shirane K et al. De novo DNA methylation drives 5hmC accumulation in mouse zygotes. *Nat Cell Biol*. 2016;18(2):225–33.

27. Peat JR, Dean W, Clark SJ et al. Genome-wide bisulphite sequencing in zygotes identifies demethylation targets and maps the contribution of TET3 oxidation. *Cell Rep*. 2014;9(6):1990–2000.

28. Lee MT, Bonneau AR, Giraldez AJ. Zygotic genome activation during the maternal-to-zygotic transition. *Annu Rev Cell Dev Biol*. 2014;30:581–613.

29. Vassena R, Boué S, González-Roca E et al. Waves of early transcriptional activation and pluripotency program initiation during human preimplantation development. *Development*. 2011;138(17):3699–709.

30. Wang X, Liu D, He D et al. Transcriptome analyses of rhesus monkey preimplantation embryos reveal a reduced capacity for DNA double-strand break repair in primate oocytes and early embryos. *Genome Res*. 2017;27(4):567–79.

31. Schramm RD, Bavister BD. Onset of nucleolar and extranucleolar transcription and expression of fibrillarin in macaque embryos developing *in vitro*. *Biol Reprod*. 1999;60(3):721–8.

32. Guo F, Li L, Li J et al. Single-cell multi-omics sequencing of mouse early embryos and embryonic stem cells. *Cell Res*. 2017;27(8):967–88.

33. Canovas S, Ivanova E, García-Martínez S et al. Species-specific differences in the methylation reprogramming during early perimplantation development. *Reproduction, Fertility, and Development*. 2016;29:1.

34. Canovas S, Ivanova E, Romar R et al. DNA methylation and gene expression changes derived from assisted reproductive technologies can be decreased by reproductive fluids. *Elife*. 2017;6:e23670.

35. Reynolds L, Ward A, Caton J. Epigenetics and developmental programming in ruminants. Long-term impacts on growth and development. In: CG HRaS, editor. *Domestic Animal Biology*. 1 ed. Milton Park, UK: CRC Press/Taylor & Francis Group, 2017. 370.

36. Barlow DP. Genomic imprinting: A mammalian epigenetic discovery model. *Annu Rev Genet*. 2011;45:379–403.

37. Barker DJ. The origins of the developmental origins theory. *J Intern Med.* 2007;261(5):412–7.

38. Cooney CA, Dave AA, Wolff GL. Maternal methyl supplements in mice affect epigenetic variation and DNA methylation of offspring. *J Nutr.* 2002;132(8 Suppl.):2393S–400S.

39. Carlin J, George R, Reyes TM. Methyl donor supplementation blocks the adverse effects of maternal high fat diet on offspring physiology. *PLoS One.* 2013;8(5):e63549.

40. Smith GS, Chambers JW, Neumann AL, Ray EE, Nelson AB. Lipotropic factors for beef cattle fed high-concentrate diets. *J Anim Sci.* 1974;38(3):627–33.

41. Cho K, Choi WS, Crane CL, Park CS. Pubertal supplementation of lipotropes in female rats reduces mammary cancer risk by suppressing histone deacetylase 1. *Eur J Nutr.* 2014;53(4):1139–43.

42. Canovas S, Ross PJ. Epigenetics in preimplantation mammalian development. *Theriogenology.* 2016;86(1):69–79.

43. Canovas S, Ross PJ, Kelsey G, Coy P. DNA methylation in embryo development: Epigenetic impact of ART (assisted reproductive technologies). *BioEssays.* 2017;39(11). doi: 10.1002/bies.201700106.

44. Pérez-Cerezales S, Ramos-Ibeas P, Acuña OS et al. The oviduct: From sperm selection to the epigenetic landscape of the embryo. *Biol Reprod.* 2017;98(3):262–76.

45. Keller TE, Yi SV. DNA methylation and evolution of duplicate genes. *Proc Natl Acad Sci USA.* 2014;111(16):5932–7.

46. Laubach ZM, Perng W, Dolinoy DC, Faulk CD, Holekamp KE, Getty T. Epigenetics and the maintenance of developmental plasticity: Extending the signalling theory framework. *Biol Rev Camb Philos Soc.* 2018. doi: 10.1111/brv.12396.

47. Bartolomei MS. Genomic imprinting: Employing and avoiding epigenetic processes. *Genes Dev.* 2009;23(18):2124–33.

48. Elhamamsy AR. Role of DNA methylation in imprinting disorders: An updated review. *J Assist Reprod Genet.* 2017;34(5):549–62.

49. Lee JT, Bartolomei MS. X-inactivation, imprinting, and long noncoding RNAs in health and disease. *Cell.* 2013;152(6):1308–23.

50. Pfeifer K. Mechanisms of genomic imprinting. *Am J Hum Genet.* 2000;67(4):777–87.

51. Himes KP, Koppes E, Chaillet JR. Generalized disruption of inherited genomic imprints leads to wide-ranging placental defects and dysregulated fetal growth. *Dev Biol.* 2013;373(1):72–82.

52. McGraw S, Oakes CC, Martel J et al. Loss of DNMT1o disrupts imprinted X chromosome inactivation and accentuates placental defects in females. *PLoS Genet.* 2013;9(11):e1003873.

53. McGrath J, Solter D. Completion of mouse embryogenesis requires both the maternal and paternal genomes. *Cell.* 1984;37(1):179–83.

54. Morgan HD, Santos F, Green K, Dean W, Reik W. Epigenetic reprogramming in mammals. *Hum Mol Genet.* 2005;14(Spec No 1):R47–58.

55. Cirio MC, Ratnam S, Ding F, Reinhart B, Navara C, Chaillet JR. Preimplantation expression of the somatic form of Dnmt1 suggests a role in the inheritance of genomic imprints. *BMC Dev Biol.* 2008;8:9.

56. Kurihara Y, Kawamura Y, Uchijima Y et al. Maintenance of genomic methylation patterns during preimplantation development requires the somatic form of DNA methyltransferase 1. *Dev Biol.* 2008;313(1):335–46.

57. Li Y, Sasaki H. Genomic imprinting in mammals: Its life cycle, molecular mechanisms and reprogramming. *Cell Res.* 2011;21(3):466–73.

58. Nakamura T, Liu YJ, Nakashima H et al. PGC7 binds histone H3K9me2 to protect against conversion of 5mC to 5hmC in early embryos. *Nature*. 2012;486(7403):415–9.

59. Reese KJ, Lin S, Verona RI, Schultz RM, Bartolomei MS. Maintenance of paternal methylation and repression of the imprinted H19 gene requires MBD3. *PLoS Genet*. 2007;3(8):e137.

60. Li X, Ito M, Zhou F et al. A maternal-zygotic effect gene, Zfp57, maintains both maternal and paternal imprints. *Dev Cell*. 2008;15(4):547–57.

61. Nakamura T, Arai Y, Umehara H et al. PGC7/Stella protects against DNA demethylation in early embryogenesis. *Nat Cell Biol*. 2007;9(1):64–71.

62. Wu MY, Tsai TF, Beaudet AL. Deficiency of Rbbp1/Arid4a and Rbbp1l1/Arid4b alters epigenetic modifications and suppresses an imprinting defect in the PWS/AS domain. *Genes Dev*. 2006;20(20):2859–70.

63. Inoue A, Jiang L, Lu F, Suzuki T, Zhang Y. Maternal H3K27me3 controls DNA methylation-independent imprinting. *Nature*. 2017;547(7664):419–24.

64. McClintock B. The origin and behavior of mutable loci in maize. *Proc Natl Acad Sci USA*. 1950;36(6):344–55.

65. Lander ES, Linton LM, Birren B et al. Initial sequencing and analysis of the human genome. *Nature*. 2001;409(6822):860–921.

66. Pray L. Transposons: The jumping genes. *Nature Education*. 2008;1(1):204.

67. Munoz-Lopez M, Garcia-Perez JL. DNA transposons: Nature and applications in genomics. *Curr Genomics*. 2010;11(2):115–28.

68. Bodak M, Yu J, Ciaudo C. Regulation of LINE-1 in mammals. *Biomol Concepts*. 2014;5(5): 409–28.

69. Richardson SR, Doucet AJ, Kopera HC, Moldovan JB, Garcia-Perez JL, Moran JV. The influence of LINE-1 and SINE retrotransposons on mammalian genomes. *Microbiol Spectr*. 2015;3(2):Mdna3-0061-2014.

70. Kazazian HH, Moran JV. The impact of L1 retrotransposons on the human genome. *Nat Genet*. 1998;19(1):19–24.

71. Slotkin RK, Martienssen R. Transposable elements and the epigenetic regulation of the genome. *Nat Rev Genet*. 2007;8(4):272–85.

72. Kazazian HH, Wong C, Youssoufian H, Scott AF, Phillips DG, Antonarakis SE. Haemophilia A resulting from *de novo* insertion of L1 sequences represents a novel mechanism for mutation in man. *Nature*. 1988;332(6160):164–6.

73. Miki Y, Nishisho I, Horii A et al. Disruption of the APC gene by a retrotransposal insertion of L1 sequence in a colon cancer. *Cancer Res*. 1992;52(3):643–5.

74. Richardson SR, Gerdes P, Gerhardt DJ et al. Heritable L1 retrotransposition in the mouse primordial germline and early embryo. *Genome Res*. 2017;27(8):1395–405.

75. Beraldi R, Pittoggi C, Sciamanna I, Mattei E, Spadafora C. Expression of LINE-1 retroposons is essential for murine preimplantation development. *Mol Reprod Dev*. 2006;73:9.

76. Kigami D, Minami N, Takayama H, Imai H. MuERV-L is one of the earliest transcribed genes in mouse one cell embryos. *Biol Reprod*. 2003;68:4.

77. Jachowicz JW, Bing X, Pontabry J, Bošković A, Rando OJ, Torres-Padilla ME. LINE-1 activation after fertilization regulates global chromatin accessibility in the early mouse embryo. *Nat Genet*. 2017;49(10):1502–10.

78. Lane N, Dean W, Erhardt S et al. Resistance of IAPs to methylation reprogramming may provide a mechanism for epigenetic inheritance in the mouse. *Genesis*. 2003;35:6.

79. Garcia-Perez JL, Widmann TJ, Adams IR. The impact of transposable elements on mammalian development. *Development*. 2016;143(22):4101–14.

80. Peterson CL, Laniel MA. Histones and histone modifications. *Curr Biol*. 2004;14(14):R546–51.

81. Kouzarides T. SnapShot: Histone-modifying enzymes. *Cell*. 2007;131(4):822.

82. Yan H, Zhang D, Liu H et al. Chromatin modifications and genomic contexts linked to dynamic DNA methylation patterns across human cell types. *Sci Rep*. 2015;5:8410.

83. Okada Y, Yamaguchi K. Epigenetic modifications and reprogramming in paternal pronucleus: Sperm, preimplantation embryo, and beyond. *Cell Mol Life Sci*. 2017;74(11):1957–67.

84. Zhou LQ, Dean J. Reprogramming the genome to totipotency in mouse embryos. *Trends Cell Biol*. 2015;25(2):82–91.

85. Marcho C, Cui W, Mager J. Epigenetic dynamics during preimplantation development. *Reproduction*. 2015;150(3):R109–20.

86. Burton A, Torres-Padilla ME. Chromatin dynamics in the regulation of cell fate allocation during early embryogenesis. *Nat Rev Mol Cell Biol*. 2014;15(11):723–34.

87. Xu Q, Xie W. Epigenome in early mammalian development: Inheritance, reprogramming, and establishment. *Trends Cell Biol*. 2017;28(3):237–53.

88. Liu X, Gao Q, Li P et al. UHRF1 targets DNMT1 for DNA methylation through cooperative binding of hemi-methylated DNA and methylated H3K9. *Nat Commun*. 2013;4:1563.

89. Rothbart SB, Dickson BM, Ong MS et al. Multivalent histone engagement by the linked tandem Tudor and PHD domains of UHRF1 is required for the epigenetic inheritance of DNA methylation. *Genes Dev*. 2013;27(11):1288–98.

90. Cheng J, Yang Y, Fang J et al. Structural insight into coordinated recognition of trimethylated histone H3 lysine 9 (H3K9me3) by the plant homeodomain (PHD) and tandem tudor domain (TTD) of UHRF1 (ubiquitin-like, containing PHD and RING finger domains, 1) protein. *J Biol Chem*. 2013;288(2):1329–39.

91. Arita K, Isogai S, Oda T et al. Recognition of modification status on a histone H3 tail by linked histone reader modules of the epigenetic regulator UHRF1. *Proc Natl Acad Sci USA*. 2012;109(32):12950–5.

92. Canovas S, Cibelli JB, Ross PJ. Jumonji domain-containing protein 3 regulates histone 3 lysine 27 methylation during bovine preimplantation development. *Proc Natl Acad Sci USA*. 2012;109(7):2400–5.

93. Chung N, Bogliotti YS, Ding W et al. Active H3K27me3 demethylation by KDM6B is required for normal development of bovine preimplantation embryos. *Epigenetics*. 2017;12(12):1048–56.

94. Bogdanovic O, Long SW, van Heeringen SJ et al. Temporal uncoupling of the DNA methylome and transcriptional repression during embryogenesis. *Genome Res*. 2011;21(8):1313–27.

95. Neri F, Incarnato D, Krepelova A et al. Genome-wide analysis identifies a functional association of Tet1 and Polycomb repressive complex 2 in mouse embryonic stem cells. *Genome Biol*. 2013;14(8):R91.

96. Ooi SK, Qiu C, Bernstein E et al. DNMT3L connects unmethylated lysine 4 of histone H3 to *de novo* methylation of DNA. *Nature*. 2007;448(7154):714–7.

97. Kokura K, Sun L, Bedford MT, Fang J. Methyl-H3K9-binding protein MPP8 mediates E-cadherin gene silencing and promotes tumour cell motility and invasion. *EMBO J*. 2010;29(21):3673–87.

98. Epsztejn-Litman S, Feldman N, Abu-Remaileh M et al. De novo DNA methylation promoted by G9a prevents reprogramming of embryonically silenced genes. *Nat Struct Mol Biol*. 2008;15(11):1176–83.

CHAPTER 4

Epigenetic Reprogramming of Mammalian Primordial Germ Cells

Sebastian Canovas and Susana M. Chuva de Sousa Lopes

CONTENTS

4.1 PGC SPECIFICATION *IN VIVO*

Primordial germ cells (PGCs) are the founder population of the germline, from which the gametes (oocytes and spermatozoa) arise. Hence, they are responsible for the transmission of genetic information from one generation to the next in order to perpetuate the species. PGCs are specified in the early post-implantation embryo and this process is characterized by three extraordinary features: (i) the place of origin of the germ cells is distant from where they mature to gametes, which entails a tightly regulated migration process to reach the gonadal ridges; (ii) the germ cells go through complex genome-wide transcriptional dynamics and epigenetic reprogramming with the purpose to form **oogonia** in the ovary or **prospermatogonia** in the testis; (iii) the germ cells undergo meiosis, a process that generates genetic variability in the mature (haploid) gametes. Any defects during germ cell formation and/or migration will compromise the persistence of the specie or limit its evolution.

In mammals, **epigenesis (or induction)** is the used mode of germ cell formation, meaning that all the epiblast cells of the young embryo have the potential to become germ cells, but only some cells (in the right place at the right time) will receive the necessary inductive signals to do so, whereas all other epiblast cells remain somatic. In mice, germline specification begins in the posterior-proximal epiblast, around E6.25 (1), with the induction of PGCs precursors (pPGCs). pPGC origin from a small founder population of 6 cells placed in the posterior-proximal epiblast, which proliferate to form a cluster of about 40 cells, held together by E-cadherin (2). The pPGCs undergo two several key events before they become lineage restricted at E7.25 (3), including repression of genes that regulate somatic cell fate and re-acquisition of expression of pluripotency genes (1,4–8). Subsequently, they migrate through the gut and dorsal mesentery to colonize the genital ridges. After gonad colonization, female (XX) PGCs continue to proliferate and enter meiosis at embryonic day (E)12.5, being subsequently arrested at diplotene stage of prophase I of meiosis and remain so until puberty. In males, PGCs undergo mitotic arrest at E13.5 and remain quiescent until shortly after birth. In humans, the timing of PGC specification is unknown, but PGCs are visible in the dorsal part of the yolk sac endoderm in embryos with 13 somites (9). It has been speculated that PGC specification in humans occurs between 12 and 16 days post fertilization (dpf) (corresponding to week 2 of development; week 4 of gestation) (10). Mouse and human PGCs show similarities and differences that will be explored along this chapter.

In mice, bone morphogenetic proteins (BMP) and WNT ligands act as inductive signals to induce the expression of the PR domain zinc-finger protein 1 PRDM1 (or BLIMP1), the earliest and indispensable factor for pPGC specification in mouse (1,6) (Figures 4.1 and 4.2). BMP4 and BMP8b from the extraembryonic ectoderm, together with BMP2 from the visceral endoderm, act coordinately to provide sufficient levels of BMP-SMAD signals to the proximal epiblast, which favors cells placed in that location to adopt a germline phenotype (11). WNT3 and nodal, which appear in the posterior epiblast at E5.5, act as key factors in those cells to respond to BMP. In the absence of WNT3 expression in knockout mice, BMP4 is still expressed in the extraembryonic ectoderm, but PRDM1 and PRDM14, another key pPGC specification factor, are not expressed (12). In addition, T (or Brachyury), a mesodermal factor induced by WNT3-β-catenin signaling is required and sufficient to sustain PRDM1 and PRDM14 expression during pPGC specification in mouse (13) (Figure 4.1). PRDM1 is necessary for repressing the somatic program during

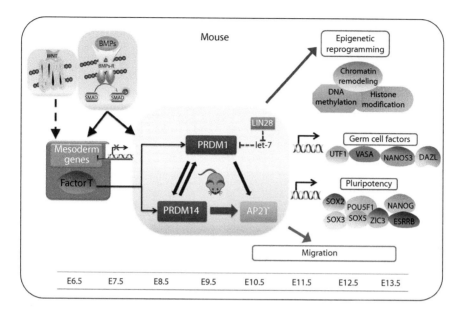

FIGURE 4.1   Transcriptional regulatory networks during mouse PGC specification.

the transition from pPGCs to PGCs and together with PRDM14, they participate in the upregulation of germ cell and pluripotency genes (4,14). In addition, nodal signaling is also considered crucial in mouse since BMP4 and WNT3 are absent in nodal null embryos (15). TCFAP2C (or AP2Υ) is another transcription factor that plays an important role in the formation of pPGCs in mice, because TCFAP2C knockout embryos contain no PGCs, both males and females (5). TCFAP2C is subjected to regulation by PRDM1 during the transition from pPGC of PGC and participates in the suppression of the genes of differentiation toward mesoderm. PRDM1, PRDM14, and TCFAP2C form a critical network to suppress the somatic program during PGC specification in mice. LIN28 is another factor involved in the initial phases during the formation of PGC. It acts by inducing the expression of PRDM1 indirectly, by inhibiting the maturation of Let-7, a microRNA that binds to PRDM1 and blocks its expression (16).

4.2 MAIN SPECIES-SPECIFIC DIFFERENCES DURING GERM CELL FORMATION BETWEEN MICE AND HUMANS

The existing knowledge about mammalian gametogenesis derives mostly from studies in mice. Nonetheless, recently studies using RNA sequencing technologies that require few cells for analysis have provided extensive transcriptional datasets of fetal human PGCs and have shed some light on the molecular mechanisms that take place during human gametogenesis (17,18). Early (migratory) PGCs share a set of key factors, such as PRDM1 and

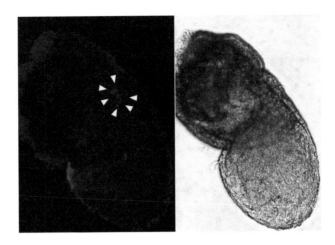

FIGURE 4.2 Mouse primordial germ cells at embryonic day 7.5 (E7.5) in transgenic mouse (PRDM1—red fluorescent protein).

TCFAP2C and pluripotency markers, including POU5F1 (or OCT4), NANOG, DPPA3 (or STELLA/PPG7), and LIN28A (Figures 4.1 and 4.3). Some late (pre-meiotic) PGC markers are also shared between the human and mouse, including the germ cell-specific UTF1, DDX4 (or VASA), NANOS3, and DAZL.

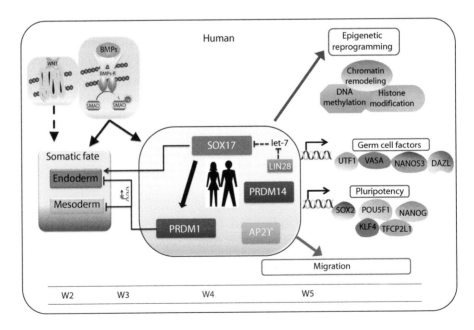

FIGURE 4.3 Transcriptional regulatory networks during human PGC specification.

Moreover, human and mouse gametogenesis differ considerably regarding morphogenesis (19). Around week (W)10–11 of development, the ovary starts to develop a strong heterogeneity regarding the composition of germ cells. Until W10, all germ cells express POU5F1 and NANOS3, but thereafter some germ cells downregulate POU5F1 and NANOS3 (early pre-meiotic markers) and upregulate DDX4 and DAZL (late pre-meiotic markers). Interestingly, this heterogeneity is spatially regulated with the peripheral rim of POU5F1 and NANOS3 germ cells becoming thinner as gestation progresses. Around W14, VASA-positive germ cells progressively enter meiosis and around W16-20, the ovary is composed of primordial follicles, germ cells in different stages of meiosis, pre-meiotic DDX4-positive germ cells and an outer rim of POU5F1-positive germ cell. In males, this heterogeneity is less pronounced, as only two types of pre-meiotic germ cells can be observed during development (DDX4-positive or POU5F1-positive germ cells). Interestingly, those can be observed side-by-side in the same seminiferous tubule (20–22).

In humans, migratory hPGCs (W4-5) lack some pluripotency factors that are strongly expressed in migratory mPGCs (ESRRB, SOX2, SOX3, ZIC3). Conversely, hPGCs show high expression of the pluripotency factors KLF4 and TFCP2L1, as well as SOX17, which are absent in mPGCs (23). It is noteworthy that in humans SOX17 works upstream of PRDM1 and presumably acts as a master regulator during hPGC specification, while in mice it seems dispensable (24–26). In humans, PRDM1 plays a role in the repression of endodermal genes that otherwise would be induced by SOX17 (Figure 4.3). Moreover, PRDM1 participates in the initial global DNA demethylation by repression of DNMT3B (23,27). In contrast, PRDM14, another key factor in mPGCs that is involved in the suppression of DNA methylation, is dispensable for hPGC development (28). PRDM14 is upregulated later in hPGCs than in mPGCs, and it is downstream of PRDM1 (24). TCFAP2C has also been identified in human PGCs and gonocytes, and is involved in testicular carcinoma *in situ* and testicular germ cell tumors (29), but its function during the formation of human PGCs is currently unknown.

4.3 EPIGENETIC REPROGRAMMING IN PGCS

Genome-Wide DNA Methylation Dynamics

In mammals, there are two major phases of epigenetic reprogramming during development. The first phase occurs in the whole embryo during preimplantation and the second phase is specific to PGCs and it takes place between specification and meiotic entry. The second phase entails a more drastic wave of DNA demethylation that affects even imprinted genes and repetitive elements, which escaped DNA demethylation during the first phase (30,31). The aim of the first phase of epigenome resetting is to replace the specific marks (except the imprints) of the unipotent and transcriptionally silent gametes by marks of totipotent diploid cells, as such that the embryo can activate its genome (embryonic genome activation) and give rise to a whole organism. In the second phase, the aim is to remove the differential parental marks in diploid PGCs, so that they can be replaced by either female-only or male-only epigenetic marks depending of the sex of the gametes to be formed. Nonetheless, specific methylated loci escape DNA demethylation and have been related with the transmission of epigenetic information to next generations (transgenerational **epigenetic inheritance**). DNA demethylation in germ cells occurs with the participation of three overlapping mechanisms: Passive replication-dependent loss of 5-methylcytosine (5mC), conversion to 5-hydroxymethylcytosine (5hmC) coupled with passive depletion, and active demethylation by repair pathways (Figure 4.4).

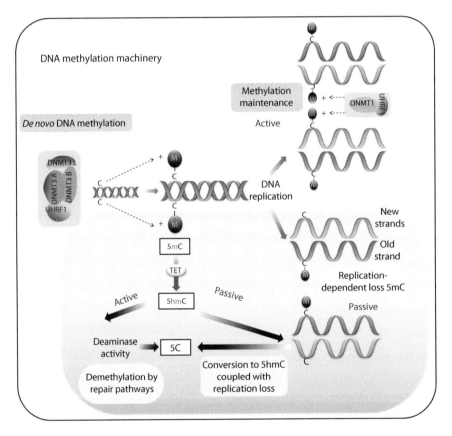

FIGURE 4.4 DNA methylation mechanisms during PGC specification. After cell DNA replication, DNMTs can recognize hemimethylated strands and methylate the new strand with the same pattern (top). In absence of DNMT activity, the new strand of DNA remains unmethylated (bottom). In addition, *de novo* DNA methylation by DNMT3A/B and hydroximethylation demethylation by TET have been reported.

In mouse germ cells, genome-wide passive DNA demethylation starts around E7.5 and it entails a initial drastic drop in levels of CpG methylation, followed by a gradual further drop during the migratory phase of the PGCs (between E7.5-10), a period during which PGCs undergo several cells divisions. This occurs in the absence of *de novo* methylation and it affects the bulk of the genome, whereas specific regions that are partially resistant, remain highly methylated until PGCs enter the genital ridges (E10). During this migratory period, a transient loss or repression of *de novo* methyltransferases (DNMT3A, DNMT3B) occurs in PGCs (14). Regarding the DNA maintenance machinery, DNMT1 is expressed in germ cells between E7.5-10, but its critical cofactor NP95 (also known as UHRF1) is localized to the cytoplasm, resulting in a disabled DNMT1 (14,32,33). Thus, the predominant mechanism of DNA demethylation during PGC migration is passive, although concomitantly DNMT1 (with the collaboration of UHRF2) and non-canonical pathway maintain methylation of specific DNA sequences (Intracisternal A-particle –IAP- elements, retroelements) (34–36).

In addition to the passive DNA demethylation by dilution during replication, the cytosine deaminases AID and APOBEC1 have been involved in genome-wide demethylation during PGC formation. These deaminases convert 5mC to thymine by deamination, creating T:G mismatches, which would become targets of glycosylases for base-excision mismatch repair (BER) (Figure 4.4). AID and BER-deficient mice show a significant increase in genome-wide DNA methylation in PGCs, which suggests that it is not loci-specific (37,38).

After the first phase of genome-wide demethylation (E7.5-10), a second wave of demethylation is observed, once PGCs reach the genital ridges (E10.5-13.5). This affects specific loci reaching almost undetectable methylation levels (around 5%) at E13.5 (39,40) (Figure 4.4). These loci include differentially methylated regions (DMR) of imprinted genes, the silent X chromosome and genes related with meiosis and gamete generation. The ten-eleven translocation enzymes TET1 and TET2, responsible for the enzymatic oxidation of 5mC to 5hmC, are implicated in locus-specific demethylation of genomic imprints, genes that regulate activation of meiotic programme in females (41), and specific germline genes such as *Dazl*, *Mael*, or *Sycp3* (42). Nonetheless, this last drop in DNA methylation levels can also happen in the absence of TET1 and TET2 (36,42).

In human migratory PGCs (W4-5), the overall DNA demethylation process seems similar to the dynamic in mouse (E7.5-10). The second wave of DNA demethylation takes place between W5.5-11 (Figure 4.5) (17,23,43).

Even though PGCs undergo two DNA demethylation waves, some specific DNA sequences seem to be **resistant DNA demethylation** ("escapees"). In the mouse, IAP retrotransposon, with mutagenic activity, are the most frequently identified demethylation-resistant regions, but there are also other sequences, such as rare retroelements (LTR-ERV1), single-copy sequences and some variable erased CpG islands (VEC) that remain methylated at all times during the life cycle. In addition, transposable elements such as long

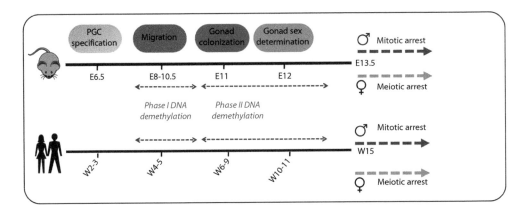

FIGURE 4.5 Timeline of main events during mouse and human PGC specification.

and short interspersed nuclear elements (LINE1s and SINEs) also retain low levels of DNA methylation. This suggests that specific regulatory mechanisms are in place to maintain loci with the potential to alter genome stability methylated (silent). In humans, "escapee" regions can "jump" and integrate randomly in regions of the genome, overlaping with gene bodies, enhancers, or promoters. Interestingly, several loci associated with metabolic and neurological disorders have been identified as resistant to DNA demethylation. In this case, these acquired epimutations can results in transgenerational inheritance resulting in transmission of the phenotype to the progeny (23,36,44,45).

After PGC specification, the majority of promoters become hypomethylated, but this is not directly associated with general transcriptional activation of the respective downstream genes (17,23,43). For further transcriptional regulation, additional mechanisms, such as the remodeling of histone modifications or incorporation of alternative histone variants, are triggered to modulate gene expression.

Ultimately, male and female (diploid) germ cells have to acquire the epigenetic marks characteristic of only the (haploid) male or only the (haploid) female gametes. Therefore, they undergo sex-specific *de novo* DNA methylation. In male mice, this reacquisition of DNA methylation starts between E14.5-16.5 and seems be completed at birth (46,47). In female mice, *de novo* DNA methylation is resumed in the first two weeks after birth (48,49).

As heterogeneity (different stages of PGC development present in the same gonad) has not been taken into account in the recent studies reporting DNA methylation in human PGCs, it is unclear whether there is DNA remethylation of some specific genomic features of whether latent DNA methylation levels reflect still ongoing demethylation in the POU5F1-positive germ cells that remain in the gonads (17,23,43). Future studies using either single-cell DNA methylation analysis or FACS sorting of pure populations of PGCs prior to methylation analysis with resolve this issue.

The re-establishment of 5mC in PGCs requires the *de novo* DNA methylation machinery, including DNMT3A and DNMT3B. However, both PIWIL and piwi-interacting RNAs (piRNAs) have also been also involved in the *de novo* methylation of transposable elements and have recently been characterized in human germ cells at different developmental stages and time points during gestation (50,51).

Histone Variants and Histone Modification Dynamics

At E6.5 mouse pPGCs show histone marks similar to the surrounding somatic cells. Main changes in histone marks start at E7 with the decrease of H3K9me1 and H3K9me2 while H3K9me3 is retained at **pericentric heterochromatin** and it is followed by a significant increase of the repressive marks H3K27me3 and H2A/H4R3me2s at E8.25 (7,8) (Figure 4.6). PRDM1 and PRMD14 repress histone methyltransferase EHMT1, which participates in the methylation of H3K9. Meanwhile, the increase in the levels of H3K27me3 is probably due to EZH2 activity, an H3K27me3 methyltransferase, which is stably expressed in PGCs at E8.25 (7,8,52). Alternatively, this could be also the result of the observed downregulation of the H3K27me3 demethylases UTX and JMJD3 (53). Other repressive histone marks, such as H2A/H4R3me2s are conferred by PRMT5, a protein arginine methyltransferase that at E8.5 in PGC translocates to the nucleus to form a complex with PRDM1.

After mPGCs arrive to the genital ridges the complex PRDM1/PRMT5 translocates from the nucleus to the cytoplasm becoming disabled and this leads to a decrease in the levels of H2A/H4R3me2s (54). In human tumoral germinal cells, PRDM1/PRMT5 does not translocate to the cytoplasm and there aberrant levels of H4/H2AR3me2S are observed (55). Moreover, gonadal mPGCs show signs of histone replacement, as rapid loss of linker

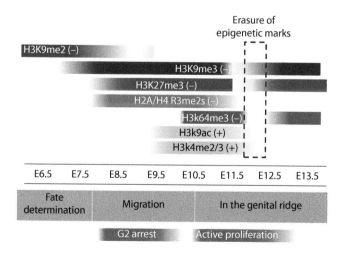

FIGURE 4.6   Histone tail modifications during mouse PGC development.

histone H1, accompanied by "loosening" of the chromatin and by an increased size of the nuclei. The levels of repressive H3K9me3, H3K27me3, and H3K64me3 transiently decline and are re-elevated afterward. There is also a loss of H3K9ac, H4/H2AR3me2s5, and histone variant H2AZ (52,56,57).

In humans, the overall reorganization of histone modifications in PGCs follows a similar dynamics to those observed in mPGCs, with slight differences regarding H3K27me3 (58). In mPGCs, there is a gradual increase in H3K27me3 from E8–13.5 (59,60) culminating with strong localization to the nuclear lamina at E13.5–15.5, when the DNA methylation levels are at their lowest (61). In humans, hPGCs show high levels of nuclear H3K27me3 in POU5F1-positive germ cells, but as they downregulate POU5F1 and upregulate DDX4, PGCs loose the H3K27me3 marks in both sexes (58).

Dynamics of X Chromosome Activity

Mammalian female and male cells have different sex chromosomes, XX and XY, respectively. The mechanism that has evolved to equalize the transcriptional levels of X-linked genes in both sexes is known as **dosage compensation**. In mammals, that is achieved by silencing one of the X chromosomes in female cells (62–65). This is a female-specific silencing mechanism that in mice takes place during preimplantation (X chromosome inactivation) (64).

In the sperm, the paternal genome is tightly wrapped around protamines even though specific regions remain packaged with histones (66,67). The protamines are rapidly exchanged by canonical histones in the zygote. At the 2-cell stadium, mice embryos activate their own genome (embryonic genome activation) and both the maternal and paternal X chromosomes are transiently active. However, at the 4-cell stage the paternal X chromosome is obligatory silenced in all cells (**imprinted X inactivation**), by a mechanism that is regulated by the long-non coding RNA *Xist*. This molecule is transcribed and binds *in cis* to the X chromosome to be silenced, first coating the region of the X chromosome close to its locus, known as the X inactivation center, and then spreading in both directions. *Xist* attracts the polycomb repressive complex 2 (PRC2), containing EZH2 and EED. There, EZH2 converts H3K27me2 to H3K27me3 silencing that X chromosome (Xi). Subsequently, Xi is maintained by incorporation of the histone variant macroH2A and gain of chromosome-wide DNA methylation (68,69).

When the mouse embryo reaches the blastocyst stage (E3.5), the cells of the inner cell mass (ICM), express a combination of pluripotency genes (*Pou5f1, Nanog, Sox2*), that bind the *Xist* promoter/exon1 silencing it (70). In addition, POUF51 and ZFP42 (or REX1) upregulate the long non-coding *Tsix*, antisense of *Xist*. Subsequently *Tsix* and *Xist* dimerize forming a double-strand that is targeted for degradation via the RNAi machinery (71). Hence, *Xist* is downregulated and the silent X chromosome is reactivated. Half a day later (E4.0), each ICM cell undergoes X chromosome inactivation again, this time **random**

X inactivation. Prior to implantation, mouse blastocysts are formed by ICM cells (with random X inactivation) and extraembryonic (trophectoderm and primitive endoderm) cells (with imprinted X inactivation). The Xi is transmitted to the daughter cells by mitosis and so the female embryo develops as mosaic, showing clonal expansion of cells with either a maternal or paternal Xi.

Before meiosis, the Xi in female mPGCs needs to be reactivated to equalize the two XX chromosomes, allowing recombination to take place. This reprogramming of the Xi that will lead to its reactivation is initiated during migration (XIST coating is removed, H3K27me3 marks are removed and DNA methylation is removed, but there is no robust expression from the Xi). It is only prior to meiosis that robust X-linked biallelic expression is detected (59,60).

In humans, the process of dosage compensation and dynamics of X chromosome regulation is not very well described. There is increasing evidence that humans do not show imprinted X inactivation and that, in contrast to mice, X inactivation does not take place during preimplantation in humans (62,72,73). Rather, it seems to take place during the peri-implantation period (74) as random X inactivation (75). Moreover, in humans the long non-coding RNA *XACT* seems to play an important role in the X inactivation mechanism, together with *XIST* (72). In addition, the exclusive role of H3K27me3 coating the Xi in mouse cells, is not observed in human cells where non-overlapping domains of H3K27me3 (and macroH2A) and H3K9me3 (and HP1) coat adjacent regions of the Xi (76).

Human female early pre-meiotic (POU5F1-positive) PGCs show basically no accumulation of H3K27me3, compared to surrounding somatic cells that have strong perinuclear localization of H3K27me3, corresponding to the Xi (or Barr body) (17,58). Nevertheless, robust biallelic expression has not been reported (17) and hence the timing of X reactivation in humans, in particular due to the increasing levels of heterogeneity in the female gonads, remains unclear.

Erasure and Acquisition of Genomic Imprints

Genomic imprinting is a mechanism that has evolved to differentiate, through sex-specific epigenetic marks at specific imprinted loci, the maternal from the paternal genomic complement. As a result, in diploid cells, the imprinted genes are only expressed from either the maternal or paternal allele (but not from both). A (diploid) embryo is only viable if it has matching maternal and paternal contribution and so combining the genetic material from two paternal or two maternal gametes does not result in a viable embryo (77,78). The mechanisms responsible for setting-up the parental-specific genomic imprints during gametogenesis (after birth in oocytes; and just prior to birth in prospermatogonia) are not well understood, even in mice (79).

Germ cells prior to meiotic entry (in females) or mitotic arrest (in males) undergo complete erasure of imprints to equalize the maternal and paternal genomic complement. Further on during gametogenesis, the haploid germ cells acquire exclusively the maternal imprinting pattern in females and the exact complementary imprinting pattern in males.

During preimplantation when genome-wide DNA demethylation is taking place in the embryo, the genomic imprinting marks are faithfully inherited through mitosis, marking the parental origin of each chromosome. Two proteins, DPPA3 and ZFP57, have been shown to be involved in the maintenance of imprints during the preimplantation period (80–82). Recruitment of ZFP57 to the imprints is associated with enrichment for H3K9me2/3 (83).

There are about 200 imprinted genes, usually (but not always) clustered in small groups (±20 separate clusters), spread throughout the genome (79). Those clusters of imprinted genes are often regulated by an (also imprinted) imprinting control region (ICR). Interestingly, each imprinted gene cluster contains both paternally expressed and maternally expressed genes as well as one (regulatory) non-coding RNA (84). Parental-specific gene silencing is achieved by differential DNA methylation of proximal promoters or intronic promoters; whereas ICRs exhibit an unusual high concentration of methylated CpGs (**CpG island**) and are mostly silenced by differential DNA methylation, but can be also be regulated by differential accumulation of repressive histone marks (85).

The timing of erasure of genomic imprints in mPGCs (and hPGCs) differs per cluster, but erasure initiates after E9.5 and is practically complete by E13.5 (40,42,86). Interestingly, when the imprinting marks are erased from the ICR region, and depending whether the ICR is maternally or paternally methylated, and whether the imprinted genes under the regulation of that particular ICR are maternally or paternally methylated, some genes of that respective cluster become biallelically expressed, whereas others are shut down completely (79,85,87).

The mechanisms used for imprint erasure (passive versus active) in mPGCs are still a matter of debate (79). Increasingly sensitive technology becoming available and affordable (methylation at single cell level or even combined methylation/transcriptome at single cell level) will help resolve this issue.

In mice, DNMT3A, DNMT3B, and DNMT3L are key regulators of *de novo* acquisition of imprints, but seem to prefer different imprinted clusters. Moreover, the timing for the acquisition on the sex-specific imprints in (the still diploid) germ cells seems to depend on parental origin of the allele (46,48,88), so even though there has been erasure of most epigenetic marks, germ cells can still recognize the parental origin. As with imprint erasure, the acquisition of imprints in mice is also cluster specific (79) and therefore it is difficult to generalize. All together, genomic imprinting adds a tremendous level of complexity to the development of germ cells during the entire gametogenesis period to ensure the generation of functional gametes.

4.4 STRATEGIES TO MODEL PGC FORMATION *IN VITRO*

In mice, it is possible to produce viable and fertile chimeras 100%-derived from pluripotent stem cells (PSCs), both from embryonic stem cells (ESCs) and induced pluripotent stem cells (iPSCs). These experiments have demonstrated that mPSCs have the potential to give rise to functionally mature gametes, provided they are exposed to the correct microenvironment. It has proved challenging to reproduce the entire cycle of gamete formation from PSCs *in vitro*. However, two recent cornerstone papers have successfully produced mouse mature gametes both female and male from PSCs, using a two-step protocol combining the early induction to PGC-like cells (PGCLCs) with co-culture with either E12.5 fetal ovaries or newborn testis to induce meiosis (89,90). These promising results are an exciting step forward to develop models to recapitulate gametogenesis entirely *in vitro*, without the need of a co-culture system using gonadal material.

In humans, the differentiation of human PGCLCs from PSCs has been successfully reported and those PGCLCs resemble early pre-meiotic PGCs (POU5F1-positive) regarding epigenetics and transcription (24,27,91). One of the reasons why the generation of PGCLCs from PSCs has proved more challenging in humans than in mice is because there are fundamental differences in the pluripotency stage of mouse PSCs (naïve stage) and human PSCs (primed stage) (24,92,93). Attempts to bring human PSCs to a more naïve stage before the induction of PGCLCs proved crucial to differentiate PGCLCs. Interestingly, hESC lines derived in the presence of Activin A seem to be able to differentiate further, to late pre-meiotic PGCs (94).

Finally, the recent success using transdifferentiation or direct conversion between different cell types (95) opens the interesting possibility of using somatic cells directly as a source to generate PGCLCs. Two studies have shown that somatic cells can be induced to express early PGC markers and resemble immature PGCLCs (96,97). As we gain more knowledge on the necessary signals to induce meiosis and how to further mature germ cells into functional gametes, protocols will keep being optimized to ultimately produce patient-specific artificial gametes.

ACKNOWLEDGMENTS

The authors thank the funding received from the Regional Agency of Science (Fundacion Seneca), Murcia, Spain (Grant 20040/GERM/16) to SC and by the European Research Council Consolidator (ERC-CoG-725722-OVOGROWTH) to SMCSL.

REFERENCES

1. Ohinata Y, Payer B, O'Carroll D et al. Blimp1 is a critical determinant of the germ cell lineage in mice. *Nature*. 2005;436(7048):207–13.

2. Di Carlo A, De Felici M. A role for E-cadherin in mouse primordial germ cell development. *Dev Biol.* 2000;226(2):209–19.

3. Tam PP, Zhou SX. The allocation of epiblast cells to ectodermal and germ-line lineages is influenced by the position of the cells in the gastrulating mouse embryo. *Dev Biol.* 1996;178(1):124–32.

4. Yamaji M, Seki Y, Kurimoto K et al. Critical function of Prdm14 for the establishment of the germ cell lineage in mice. *Nat Genet.* 2008;40(8):1016–22.

5. Weber S, Eckert D, Nettersheim D et al. Critical function of AP-2 gamma/TCFAP2C in mouse embryonic germ cell maintenance. *Biol Reprod.* 2010;82(1):214–23.

6. Vincent SD, Dunn NR, Sciammas R et al. The zinc finger transcriptional repressor Blimp1/Prdm1 is dispensable for early axis formation but is required for specification of primordial germ cells in the mouse. *Development.* 2005;132(6):1315–25.

7. Seki Y, Hayashi K, Itoh K, Mizugaki M, Saitou M, Matsui Y. Extensive and orderly reprogramming of genome-wide chromatin modifications associated with specification and early development of germ cells in mice. *Dev Biol.* 2005;278(2):440–58.

8. Seki Y, Yamaji M, Yabuta Y et al. Cellular dynamics associated with the genome-wide epigenetic reprogramming in migrating primordial germ cells in mice. *Development.* 2007;134(14):2627–38.

9. Witschi E. Migration of germ cells of human embryos from the yolk sac to the primitive gonadal folds. *Contrib Embryol Carnegie Inst.* 1948;209:67–98.

10. Leitch HG, Tang WW, Surani MA. Primordial germ-cell development and epigenetic reprogramming in mammals. *Curr Top Dev Biol.* 2013;104:149–87.

11. de Sousa Lopes SM, Roelen BA, Monteiro RM et al. BMP signaling mediated by ALK2 in the visceral endoderm is necessary for the generation of primordial germ cells in the mouse embryo. *Genes Dev.* 2004;18(15):1838–49.

12. Ohinata Y, Ohta H, Shigeta M, Yamanaka K et al. A signaling principle for the specification of the germ cell lineage in mice. *Cell.* 2009;137(3):571–84.

13. Aramaki S, Hayashi K, Kurimoto K et al. A mesodermal factor, T, specifies mouse germ cell fate by directly activating germline determinants. *Dev Cell.* 2013;27(5):516–29.

14. Kurimoto K, Yamaji M, Seki Y, Saitou M. Specification of the germ cell lineage in mice: A process orchestrated by the PR-domain proteins, Blimp1, and Prdm14. *Cell Cycle.* 2008;7(22):3514–8.

15. Brennan J, Lu CC, Norris DP, Rodriguez TA et al. Nodal signalling in the epiblast patterns the early mouse embryo. *Nature.* 2001;411(6840):965–9.

16. West JA, Viswanathan SR, Yabuuchi A et al. A role for Lin28 in primordial germ-cell development and germ-cell malignancy. *Nature.* 2009;460(7257):909–13.

17. Guo F, Yan L, Guo H et al. The transcriptome and DNA methylome landscapes of human primordial germ cells. *Cell.* 2015;161(6):1437–52.

18. Li L, Dong J, Yan L et al. Single-cell RNA-Seq analysis maps development of human germline cells and gonadal niche interactions. *Cell Stem Cell.* 2017;20(6):891–2.

19. Bertocchini F, Chuva de Sousa Lopes SM. Germline development in amniotes: A paradigm shift in primordial germ cell specification. *Bioessays.* 2016;38(8):791–800.

20. Heeren AM, He N, de Souza AF et al. On the development of extragonadal and gonadal human germ cells. *Biol Open.* 2016;5(2):185–94.

21. Heeren AM, van Iperen L, Klootwijk DB et al. Development of the follicular basement membrane during human gametogenesis and early folliculogenesis. *BMC Dev Biol.* 2015;15:4.

22. Anderson RA, Fulton N, Cowan G et al. Conserved and divergent patterns of expression of DAZL, VASA, and OCT4 in the germ cells of the human fetal ovary and testis. *BMC Dev Biol*. 2007;7:136.

23. Tang WW, Dietmann S, Irie N et al. A unique gene regulatory network resets the human germline epigenome for development. *Cell*. 2015;161(6):1453–67.

24. Irie N, Weinberger L, Tang WW et al. SOX17 is a critical specifier of human primordial germ cell fate. *Cell*. 2015;160(1–2):253–68.

25. Magnusdottir E, Dietmann S, Murakami K et al. A tripartite transcription factor network regulates primordial germ cell specification in mice. *Nat Cell Biol*. 2013;15(8):905–15.

26. Nakaki F, Hayashi K, Ohta H, Kurimoto K et al. Induction of mouse germ-cell fate by transcription factors *in vitro*. *Nature*. 2013;501(7466):222–6.

27. Sasaki K, Yokobayashi S, Nakamura T et al. Robust *in vitro* induction of human germ cell fate from pluripotent stem cells. *Cell Stem Cell*. 2015;17(2):178–94.

28. Sugawa F, Arauzo-Bravo MJ, Yoon J et al. Human primordial germ cell commitment *in vitro* associates with a unique PRDM14 expression profile. *Embo J*. 2015;34(8):1009–24.

29. Hoei-Hansen CE, Nielsen JE, Almstrup K et al. Identification of genes differentially expressed in testes containing carcinoma *in situ*. *Mol Hum Reprod*. 2004;10(6):423–31.

30. Oswald J, Engemann S, Lane N et al. Active demethylation of the paternal genome in the mouse zygote. *Curr Biol*. 2000;10(8):475–8.

31. Mayer W, Niveleau A, Walter J et al. Demethylation of the zygotic paternal genome. *Nature*. 2000;403(6769):501–2.

32. Sharif J, Muto M, Takebayashi S et al. The SRA protein Np95 mediates epigenetic inheritance by recruiting Dnmt1 to methylated DNA. *Nature*. 2007;450(7171):908–12.

33. Ohno R, Nakayama M, Naruse C et al. A replication-dependent passive mechanism modulates DNA demethylation in mouse primordial germ cells. *Development*. 2013;140(14):2892–903.

34. Arand J, Wossidlo M, Lepikhov K et al. Selective impairment of methylation maintenance is the major cause of DNA methylation reprogramming in the early embryo. *Epigenetics Chromatin*. 2015;8(1):1.

35. Hackett JA, Surani MA. DNA methylation dynamics during the mammalian life cycle. *Philos Trans R Soc Lond B Biol Sci*. 2013;368(1609):20110328.

36. Seisenberger S, Andrews S, Krueger F et al. The dynamics of genome-wide DNA methylation reprogramming in mouse primordial germ cells. *Mol Cell*. 2012;48(6):849–62.

37. Cortellino S, Xu J, Sannai M et al. Thymine DNA glycosylase is essential for active DNA demethylation by linked deamination-base excision repair. *Cell*. 2011;146(1):67–79.

38. Popp C, Dean W, Feng S et al. Genome-wide erasure of DNA methylation in mouse primordial germ cells is affected by AID deficiency. *Nature*. 2010;463(7284):1101–5.

39. Kobayashi H, Sakurai T, Imai M et al. Contribution of intragenic DNA methylation in mouse gametic DNA methylomes to establish oocyte-specific heritable marks. *PLoS Genet*. 2012;8(1):e1002440.

40. Kobayashi H, Sakurai T, Miura F et al. High-resolution DNA methylome analysis of primordial germ cells identifies gender-specific reprogramming in mice. *Genome Res*. 2013;23(4):616–27.

41. Yamaguchi S, Hong K, Liu R et al. Tet1 controls meiosis by regulating meiotic gene expression. *Nature*. 2012;492(7429):443–7.

42. Hackett JA, Sengupta R, Zylicz JJ et al. Germline DNA demethylation dynamics and imprint erasure through 5-hydroxymethylcytosine. *Science*. 2013;339(6118):448–52.
43. Gkountela S, Zhang KX, Shafiq TA et al. DNA demethylation dynamics in the human prenatal germline. *Cell*. 2015;161(6):1425–36.
44. Guibert S, Forne T, Weber M. Global profiling of DNA methylation erasure in mouse primordial germ cells. *Genome Res*. 2012;22(4):633–41.
45. Daxinger L, Whitelaw E. Understanding transgenerational epigenetic inheritance via the gametes in mammals. *Nat Rev Genet*. 2012;13(3):153–62.
46. Davis TL, Yang GJ, McCarrey JR, Bartolomei MS. The H19 methylation imprint is erased and re-established differentially on the parental alleles during male germ cell development. *Hum Mol Genet*. 2000;9(19):2885–94.
47. Kato Y, Kaneda M, Hata K et al. Role of the Dnmt3 family in *de novo* methylation of imprinted and repetitive sequences during male germ cell development in the mouse. *Hum Mol Genet*. 2007;16(19):2272–80.
48. Lucifero D, Mann MR, Bartolomei MS, Trasler JM. Gene-specific timing and epigenetic memory in oocyte imprinting. *Hum Mol Genet*. 2004;13(8):839–49.
49. Smallwood SA, Tomizawa S, Krueger F et al. Dynamic CpG island methylation landscape in oocytes and preimplantation embryos. *Nat Genet*. 2011;43(8):811–4.
50. Roovers EF, Rosenkranz D, Mahdipour M et al. Piwi proteins and piRNAs in mammalian oocytes and early embryos. *Cell Rep*. 2015;10(12):2069–82.
51. Gomes Fernandes M, He N, Wang F et al. Human-specific subcellular compartmentalization of P-element induced wimpy testis-like (PIWIL) granules during germ cell development and spermatogenesis. *Hum Reprod*. 2017;33(2):258–69.
52. Hajkova P, Ancelin K, Waldmann T et al. Chromatin dynamics during epigenetic reprogramming in the mouse germ line. *Nature*. 2008;452(7189):877–81.
53. Mansour AA, Gafni O, Weinberger L et al. The H3K27 demethylase Utx regulates somatic and germ cell epigenetic reprogramming. *Nature*. 2012;488(7411):409–13.
54. Ancelin K, Lange UC, Hajkova P et al. Blimp1 associates with Prmt5 and directs histone arginine methylation in mouse germ cells. *Nat Cell Biol*. 2006;8(6):623–30.
55. Eckert D, Biermann K, Nettersheim D et al. Expression of BLIMP1/PRMT5 and concurrent histone H2A/H4 arginine 3 dimethylation in fetal germ cells, CIS/IGCNU and germ cell tumors. *BMC Dev Biol*. 2008;8:106.
56. Daujat S, Weiss T, Mohn F et al. H3K64 trimethylation marks heterochromatin and is dynamically remodeled during developmental reprogramming. *Nat Struct Mol Biol*. 2009;16(7):777–81.
57. Kagiwada S, Kurimoto K, Hirota T, Yamaji M, Saitou M. Replication-coupled passive DNA demethylation for the erasure of genome imprints in mice. *EMBO J*. 2013;32(3):340–53.
58. Gkountela S, Li Z, Vincent JJ et al. The ontogeny of cKIT+ human primordial germ cells proves to be a resource for human germ line reprogramming, imprint erasure and *in vitro* differentiation. *Nat Cell Biol*. 2013;15(1):113–22.
59. Chuva de Sousa Lopes SM, Hayashi K, Shovlin TC, Mifsud W, Surani MA, McLaren A. X chromosome activity in mouse XX primordial germ cells. *PLoS Genet*. 2008;4(2):e30.
60. Sugimoto M, Abe K. X chromosome reactivation initiates in nascent primordial germ cells in mice. *PLoS Genet*. 2007;3(7):e116.

61. Prokopuk L, Stringer JM, Hogg K, Elgass KD, Western PS. PRC2 is required for extensive reorganization of H3K27me3 during epigenetic reprogramming in mouse fetal germ cells. *Epigenetics Chromatin.* 2017;10:7.

62. Deng X, Berletch JB, Nguyen DK, Disteche CM. X chromosome regulation: Diverse patterns in development, tissues and disease. *Nat Rev Genet.* 2014;15(6):367–78.

63. Vallot C, Ouimette JF, Rougeulle C. Establishment of X chromosome inactivation and epigenomic features of the inactive X depend on cellular contexts. *Bioessays.* 2016;38(9):869–80.

64. Payer B, Lee JT. X chromosome dosage compensation: How mammals keep the balance. *Annu Rev Genet.* 2008;42:733–72.

65. Payer B. Developmental regulation of X-chromosome inactivation. *Semin Cell Dev Biol.* 2016;56:88–99.

66. Hammoud SS, Nix DA, Zhang H, Purwar J, Carrell DT, Cairns BR. Distinctive chromatin in human sperm packages genes for embryo development. *Nature.* 2009;460(7254):473–8.

67. Gatewood JM, Cook GR, Balhorn R, Schmid CW, Bradbury EM. Isolation of four core histones from human sperm chromatin representing a minor subset of somatic histones. *J Biol Chem.* 1990;265(33):20662–6.

68. Maduro C, de Hoon B, Gribnau J. Fitting the puzzle pieces: The bigger picture of XCI. *Trends Biochem Sci.* 2016;41(2):138–47.

69. Jeon Y, Sarma K, Lee JT. New and Xisting regulatory mechanisms of X chromosome inactivation. *Curr Opin Genet Dev.* 2012;22(2):62–71.

70. Navarro P, Chambers I, Karwacki-Neisius V et al. Molecular coupling of Xist regulation and pluripotency. *Science.* 2008;321(5896):1693–5.

71. Ogawa Y, Sun BK, Lee JT. Intersection of the RNA interference and X-inactivation pathways. *Science.* 2008;320(5881):1336–41.

72. Vallot C, Patrat C, Collier AJ et al. XACT noncoding RNA competes with XIST in the control of X chromosome activity during human early development. *Cell Stem Cell.* 2017;20(1):102–11.

73. Petropoulos S, Edsgard D, Reinius B et al. Single-cell RNA-Seq reveals lineage and X chromosome dynamics in human preimplantation embryos. *Cell.* 2016;165(4):1012–26.

74. O'Leary T, Heindryckx B, Lierman S et al. Tracking the progression of the human inner cell mass during embryonic stem cell derivation. *Nat Biotechnol.* 2012;30(3):278–82.

75. Moreira de Mello JC, de Araujo ES, Stabellini R et al. Random X inactivation and extensive mosaicism in human placenta revealed by analysis of allele-specific gene expression along the X chromosome. *PLoS One.* 2010;5(6):e10947.

76. Chadwick BP, Willard HF. Multiple spatially distinct types of facultative heterochromatin on the human inactive X chromosome. *Proc Natl Acad Sci USA.* 2004;101(50):17450–5.

77. Barton SC, Surani MA, Norris ML. Role of paternal and maternal genomes in mouse development. *Nature.* 1984;311(5984):374–6.

78. McGrath J, Solter D. Completion of mouse embryogenesis requires both the maternal and paternal genomes. *Cell.* 1984;37(1):179–83.

79. MacDonald WA, Mann MR. Epigenetic regulation of genomic imprinting from germ line to preimplantation. *Mol Reprod Dev.* 2014;81(2):126–40.

80. Nakamura T, Arai Y, Umehara H et al. PGC7/Stella protects against DNA demethylation in early embryogenesis. *Nat Cell Biol.* 2007;9(1):64–71.

81. Li X, Ito M, Zhou F et al. A maternal-zygotic effect gene, Zfp57, maintains both maternal and paternal imprints. *Dev Cell*. 2008;15(4):547–57.

82. Mackay DJ, Callaway JL, Marks SM et al. Hypomethylation of multiple imprinted loci in individuals with transient neonatal diabetes is associated with mutations in ZFP57. *Nat Genet*. 2008;40(8):949–51.

83. Quenneville S, Verde G, Corsinotti A et al. In embryonic stem cells, ZFP57/KAP1 recognize a methylated hexanucleotide to affect chromatin and DNA methylation of imprinting control regions. *Mol Cell*. 2011;44(3):361–72.

84. Lee JT, Bartolomei MS. X-inactivation, imprinting, and long noncoding RNAs in health and disease. *Cell*. 2013;152(6):1308–23.

85. Arnaud P. Genomic imprinting in germ cells: Imprints are under control. *Reproduction*. 2010;140(3):411–23.

86. Hajkova P, Erhardt S, Lane N et al. Epigenetic reprogramming in mouse primordial germ cells. *Mech Dev*. 2002;117(1–2):15–23.

87. Barlow DP. Genomic imprinting: A mammalian epigenetic discovery model. *Annu Rev Genet*. 2011;45:379–403.

88. Hiura H, Obata Y, Komiyama J, Shirai M, Kono T. Oocyte growth-dependent progression of maternal imprinting in mice. *Genes Cells*. 2006;11(4):353–61.

89. Hikabe O, Hamazaki N, Nagamatsu G et al. Reconstitution *in vitro* of the entire cycle of the mouse female germ line. *Nature*. 2016;539(7628):299–303.

90. Zhou Q, Wang M, Yuan Y et al. Complete meiosis from embryonic stem cell-derived germ cells *in vitro*. *Cell Stem Cell*. 2016;18(3):330–40.

91. Mitsunaga S, Odajima J, Yawata S et al. Relevance of iPSC-derived human PGC-like cells at the surface of embryoid bodies to prechemotaxis migrating PGCs. *Proc Natl Acad Sci USA*. 2017;114(46):E9913–E22.

92. Nichols J, Silva J, Roode M, Smith A. Suppression of Erk signalling promotes ground state pluripotency in the mouse embryo. *Development*. 2009;136(19):3215–22.

93. Nichols J, Smith A. Naive and primed pluripotent states. *Cell Stem Cell*. 2009;4(6):487–92.

94. Duggal G, Heindryckx B, Warrier S et al. Exogenous supplementation of Activin A enhances germ cell differentiation of human embryonic stem cells. *Mol Hum Reprod*. 2015;21(5):410–23.

95. Srivastava D, DeWitt N. *In vivo* cellular reprogramming: The next generation. *Cell*. 2016;166(6):1386–96.

96. Medrano JV, Martínez-Arroyo AM, Míguez JM et al. Human somatic cells subjected to genetic induction with six germ line-related factors display meiotic germ cell-like features. *Sci Rep*. 2016;6:24956.

97. Canovas S, Campos R, Aguilar E, Cibelli JB. Progress towards human primordial germ cell specification *in vitro*. *Mol Hum Reprod*. 2017;23(1):4–15.

CHAPTER 5

Laboratory Molecular Methodologies to Analyze DNA Methylation

David Monk and Gavin Kelsey

CONTENTS

5.1   INTRODUCTION

DNA methylation involves the addition of a methyl group to the fifth carbon of the DNA cytosine base (C), forming 5-methyl-cytsone (5mC). This represents one of the most studied epigenetic marks, primarily due to the fact that this modification is stable in archived DNA samples. DNA methylation predominantly occurs at CpG dinucleotides (CpGs), but in certain tissues and developmental settings it can occur in non-CpG contexts (e.g., CHG and CHH, where H = A, T, C). The process of methylating CpGs is catalyzed by the DNA methyltransferases (DNMTs), of which 3 are responsible for the *de novo* establishment, DNMT3A and DNMT3B (1) and an active rodent-specific pseudogene, DNMT3C, which is responsible for silencing retrotransposons (2). Once present, maintenance of the methylation profile during replication is performed by DNMT1 (3). DNA methylation has been associated with a number cellular processes including X chromosome inactivation in females, genomic imprinting, retrotransposon silencing and transcriptional repression, many of which show temporal profiles, highlighted by the dynamically remodeled that occurs during distinct epigenetic reprograming events (4).

DNA methylation does not only occur at cytosine bases, as methylation can also be present as N^6-methyladenine (6mA) in unicellular eukaryotes through to human, although the abundance of 6mA in the genome is much lower than 5mC (5). 5mC can be oxidized to 5-hydroxymethylcytosine (5hmC) and the further derivatives 5-formylcytosine (5fC) ad 5-carboxylcytosine (5aC) by the ten-eleven translocations (TET) enzymes (6), as one pathway for the removal of 5mC.

The distribution of DNA methylation varies across the mammalian genome. In somatic tissues, CpGs are usually highly methylated, which ensures that repetitive DNA elements remain silenced (7), whereas unmethylated CpGs are enriched in CpG islands often located within the promoter of genes. Promoter methylation is inversely correlated with transcription, presumably by altering chromatin accessibility to transcription factors and RNA polymerase. Methylated CpG-rich sequences are recognized by several methyl-CpG binding domain (MBD) containing proteins, including MBD1-4 and MeCP2 (8), while unmethylated CpG islands are bound by the CXXC finger protein, CFP1 (9) and other CXXC-domain containing proteins. However, positive correlations between active transcription and gene body methylation has been observed for highly expressed genes, the active X chromosome in females (10) and active transcription is essential for the establishment of methylation in the female germline (11).

It has been shown that methylation patterns can be altered during aging and disease. Aberrant methylation is a well-recognized hallmark in cancer, but also several other complex disorders including heart disease, diabetes, neurological disorders and infertility. Following many years of research, unique methylation signatures have been shown to serve as useful biomarkers for diagnosis, prognosis, and predicting response to therapy.

The importance of DNA methylation and the subtleties associated with CpG location would not have been revealed without advances in profiling technologies. In recent years, this has been accelerated with the development of high-density oligonucleotide arrays, with the latest version quantifying up to ~5% of total human CpG content, while next generation sequencing (NGS) allows for unprecedented coverage of any genome. In this chapter we provide an overview of the majority of methylation profiling methods utilized today, the advantages and disadvantages of each technology, which will allow readers to make an informed choice of which method best suits their needs. Finally, we introduce the most recent developments in epigenetic research, including the profiling of single cells, the quantification of the 5hmC, and the use of third-generation sequencing techniques for detecting methylation directly.

Advances in Methylation Detection

The analysis of methylation is hindered by the fact that methylation information is not retained during PCR amplifications, cloning in bacterial systems or nucleic acid probe hybridization. Early studies of DNA methylation focused on quantifying the total amount of 5mC in a sample using techniques such as single-nucleotide high-performance liquid chromatography (HPLC) (12) or liquid chromatography with tandem mass spectrometry (LC-MS) (13). The first assays, capable of detecting methylation at loci or repetitive elements, employed digestion of genomic DNA with methylation-sensitive restriction enzymes followed by Southern blotting (14) or PCR amplification. These were followed by methods designed to interrogate multiple loci, such as restriction landmark genome scanning (15) or detect methylation differences between samples, such as methylation-sensitive representation difference analysis (16) (Table 5.1). These methods vary in difficulty, with researchers often encountering problems such as the lack of informative restriction sites, incomplete digestions, and the requirement for a large amount of DNA, often in excess of 5–10 µg.

Following the pivotal publication by Frommer and colleagues in the early 1990s (17) that reported the conversion of unmethylated cytosines to uracils following exposure to sodium bisulfite, while 5mC remained intact, methods with single-base resolution started to be described. Originally, bisulfite conversion was coupled with PCR and Sanger sequencing, but more recently it has been combined with arrays and next generation sequencing (NGS) technologies. In general, candidate biomarkers and genome-wide profiling are discovered

TABLE 5.1 Techniques for Genome-Wide Methylation Analysis

Method	Description	Advantages	Disadvantages
		Restriction Enzyme-Based Methods	
RLGS	DNA digested with methylation-sensitive enzyme and two-dimensional electrophoresis.	• Methylation profiles are quantitative. • Applicable to any genome without prior knowledge of sequence.	• Original protocols employed radioactive labeling. • Sequencing of downstream targets difficult. • Not allelic.
ms-RDA	Recovery of unmethylated fragments following methylation-sensitive restriction enzyme digestion combined with a subtractive hybridization.	• Applicable to any genome without prior knowledge of sequence. • Can use different enzymes to increase coverage.	• Identification of downstream targets difficult. • Subject to PCR bias, requires extensive optimization. • Relatively low coverage. • Not allelic.
MRE-seq	Sequencing of small fragments generated from methylation-sensitive restriction enzymes digestions.	• Applicable to any genome without prior knowledge of sequence. • Can use different enzymes to increase coverage.	• Only unmethylated CpG sites within enzyme recognition sites analyzed. • Relatively low coverage.
		Affinity-Based Methods	
meDIP-seq	Single-stranded DNA immunoprecipitated with antibodies raised against methylated cytosines.	• Can be tailored to 5mC or 5hmC enrichment. • Can reveal allelic information. • Cost effective.	• Low resolution, not at individual CpG resolution. • Not quantitative, only predicts relative methylation.
MBD-seq	Pull-down of double-stranded DNA with MBD2-protein.	• Efficient at identifying methylation at CpG-dense regions. • Can discriminate 5mC and 5hmC. • Can reveal allelic information. • Cost effective.	• Low resolution. • Bias toward CpG-rich loci. • No information regarding unmethylated positions.
MIRA	Pull-down of double-stranded DNA with MBD2b/MBD3L1 complex.	• Efficient at identifying methylation at CpG-dense regions. • Can reveal allelic information. • Cost effective.	• Low resolution. • Relative bias toward CpG-rich loci. • No information regarding unmethylated positions.

(Continued)

TABLE 5.1 (*Continued*) Techniques for Genome-Wide Methylation Analysis

Method	Description	Advantages	Disadvantages
Array-Based Technologies			
Oligonucleotide arrays	Bisulfite-treated DNA is subject to limited amplifications and hybridized to array.	• Commercially available. • Downstream bioinformatics analysis well described. • Individual CpG resolution. • Applicable to FFPE-derived DNA. • Protocol adapted for 5hmC analysis. • Cost effective.	• Methylation profiling limited to specific CpGs targeted by probes. • Not allelic. • Platforms regularly updated.
Bisulfite Modification-Based Methods			
RRBS	Bisulfite sequencing of the small DNA fragments that result from Msp1 digestion.	• Cost effective compared to other bisulfite-seq methods. • Highly sensitive. • Allele and strand-specific profiles revealed. • Reveals non-CpG methylation.	• Exhibits limited coverage associated with restriction enzyme fragmentation (~5% coverage). • Standard bisulfite conversion does not discriminate 5mC and 5hmC. • Bias toward CpG-rich sequences.
Methyl-seq	Whole genome sequencing following bisulfite conversion.	• Data generated for the majority of CpGs in genome (~90% coverage). • Allele and strand-specific profiles revealed. • Reveals non-CpG methylation.	• Standard bisulfite conversion does not discriminate 5mC and 5hmC. • Very expensive. • Requires large amount of starting material. • Bioinformatically challenging.
Capture-seq	Captured of either pre- or post-bisulfite treated DNA with bait sequences followed by NGS.	• Cost effective compared to other bisulfite-seq methods. • Reduced sequencing effort as only CpG containing intervals captured (~15% coverage depending of kit). • Allele and strand-specific profiles revealed. • Reveals non-CpG methylation.	• Standard bisulfite conversion does not discriminate 5mC and 5hmC. • Requires large amount of starting material. • Bioinformatically challenging.
PBAT	Similar to methyl-seq except the adaptors are ligated after bisulfite conversion, thus taking advantage of fragmentation during chemical treatment.	• Scalable, for low input samples. • Limits sample degradation. • Allele and strand-specific profiles revealed. • Reveals non-CpG methylation.	• Standard bisulfite conversion does not discriminate 5mC and 5hmC. • Very expensive. • Bioinformatically challenging.

using large-scale methylation sequencing and/or array-based approaches, followed by validation using highly targeted locus-specific assays. While there are still challenges in effective DNA methylation-based detection, several emerging techniques quantifying 5mC and 5hmC are addressing these issues and will be discussed toward the end of this chapter.

5.2 GENOME-WIDE METHYLATION ASSESSMENT

Restriction Enzyme-Based Methods

Restriction enzyme-based methods often utilize the advantage of parallel digestion of genomic DNA samples with enzyme isoschizomers. These enzymes cut at the same base position within the identical recognition sequences but differ in their sensitivities to methylation. The most commonly used isoschizomers for methylation studies are HpaII, which only cleaves unmethylated target sequences and MspI that cuts all recognition sites irrespective of the methylation status. Genomic DNA digested with methylation-sensitive restriction enzymes (MSRE) can be incorporated into a number of methods, some designed to estimate the levels at individual loci (quantitative qPCR and allelic PCR) or for low-resolution genome-wide methylation profiling such as MRE-seq (Table 5.1, Figure 5.1). During methylation-sensitive enzyme (MRE)-seq, the restriction enzyme cuts only the unmethylated positions resulting in DNA fragments that are small enough to generate size-selected libraries for NGS, thus revealing the location of unmethylated CpG sites.

Affinity-Based Capture Techniques

Affinity-based enrichment methods lack the base-pair resolution offered by some technologies but have greater coverage than MRE-seq. Pull-down of methylated DNA fragments is possible with antibodies raised against 5mC (meDIP) or antibodies that recognize MBD proteins to enrich for methylation DNA fragments rather than giving absolute methylation levels (Table 5.1, Figure 5.1). These techniques typically offer 100–300 bp resolution (depending on sonication fragmentation) and are useful if high-resolution mapping is not required. Subsequently, the methylated fractions obtained from meDIP or MBD-precipitations can be used for locus-specific assessment using qPCR, hybridized to arrays or sequenced using NGS-technologies (Table 5.1, Figure 5.1).

There are important differences to consider when comparing meDIP or MBD-based methods. The 5mC antibodies employed for immunoprecipitation recognize single-stranded, denatured DNA, while MBD proteins bind double-stranded DNA. Comparisons of the two techniques coupled with NGS revealed that MBD methods enriched CpG-rich sequences better, while meDIP provide superior enrichment of low CpG density intervals, but both techniques are relatively poor at identifying methylation differences in CpG-poor regions (18,19). The specificity toward highly methylated DNA can be increased by

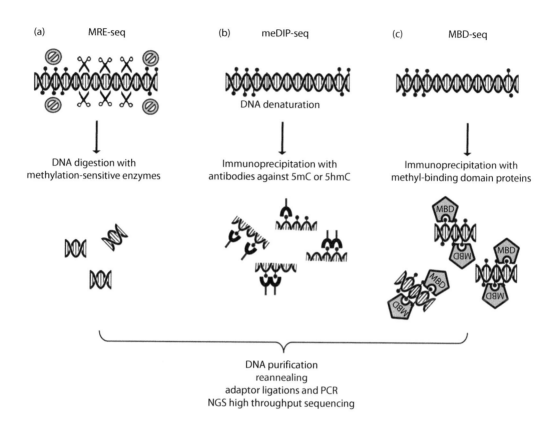

FIGURE 5.1 Genome-wide methods, not based on bisulfite conversion, for profiling DNA methylation in bulk samples. (a) MRE-seq: Several methylation-sensitive restriction enzymes can be used to digest genomic DNA. The resulting fragments are size-selected, which due to the bias toward CpG-rich loci means that smaller fragments will over-represent sequences originating from CpG islands. (b) meDIP: Genomic DNA is sheared by sonication to an average size of ~200 bp, denatured and immunoprecipitated with antibodies against 5-methylcytosine. (c) MBD-seq: Following random fragmentation of genomic DNA, methylated molecules are selected by performing MBD-capture during which all methylated fragments are collected and unmethylated DNA discarded. The resulting precipitated DNA is now suitable for downstream applications. Following the enrichment of target fragments, the DNA obtained from these three methods can be used for library preparation and NGS with the sequences mapped back to the reference assembly genome.

combining two MBD proteins in the same experiment, MBD2 and MBD3L1, in a technique referred to as methylated-CpG recovery assay, MIRA (20). However it should be noted that in many cases hypomethylation events are of particular interest and are often difficult to quantify using these methylation-enrichment based methods. Another confound in meDIP is that there is a complex, non-linear relationship between precipitation efficiency and sequence composition, so that CG density strongly influences the sensitivity of detecting methylation differences between samples.

Bisulfite Conversion-Based Methods

BeadChIPs

A major breakthrough for large-scale methylation profiling was the implementation of genotype technologies for quantifying C/T variants generated during bisulfite conversion. The most popular of the initial commercial platforms was the Illumina GoldenGate Assay that utilized multiple probes for each interrogated CpG site: Two allele-specific oligonucleotides (ASO) and two locus-specific oligonucleotides (LSO). Each ASO-LSO pair corresponded to either the methylated or unmethylated state of a CpG site and was based on methylation-specific primer design. While this platform was extremely popular and had the possibility for custom design, it had restricted multiplex capacity, limited to ~1500 sites.

Subsequently, the design and chemistries utilized by Illumina changed from GoldenGate to Infinium-bead assays. Three platforms have been released with increasing genome coverage: The HumanMethylation27 (HM27k) that was phased out in 2010, HumanMethylation450 (HM450k), which was replaced in 2016 with the MethylationEPIC array, which interrogate 27,578, 487,577, and 853,307 CpG sites, respectively. The latest version, the MethylationEPIC includes >90% of the CpGs from the HM450k design, plus an additional 413,743 CpG probes that include 350,000 sites identified as potential enhancers by FANTOM5 and the ENCODE project (21) (Table 5.1).

Each individual bead is conjugated to an oligonucleotide comprising a 23 bp address to allow identification of their physical location on the BeadChip and a 50 bp probe that is designed complementary to the bisulfite-converted DNA with a CpG site at the 3′ end of the probe. After hybridization to bisulfite converted DNA, single-base extension of the probe incorporates a fluorescently labeled ddNTP at the 3′ CpG site to allow "genotyping" of the C/T bases that result from bisulfite conversion.

The Infinium HM450k and MethylationEPIC BeadChips have two different probe designs: The Infinium type II and I. The type I probes, which originate from the HM27k design, target each CpG which two bead types, one for the methylated C and another for the unmethylated T variant, whereas the type II probes have just one probes sequence per CpG site (Figure 5.2). The performance of the two types differs slightly, with the type II probes less able to report extreme hypomethylated (<10%) and methylated (>85%) states (22), thus bioinformatics normalization is required. Both designs are deemed necessary as type I probes allow for the quantification at CpG-rich loci, whist type II probes report methylation at CpG-poor regions. Overall it has been reported that Infinium-based BeadChIP arrays are extremely reproducible with a resolution of ~2.5% and with end results highly correlated (R > 0.9) with methyl-seq quantification (23).

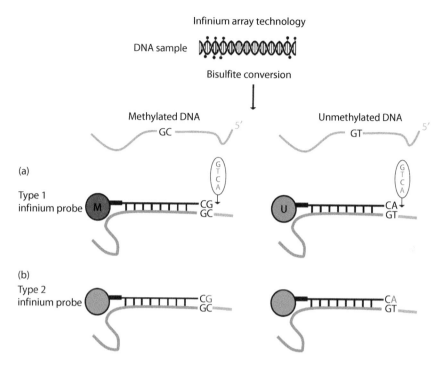

FIGURE 5.2   Probe design for the Illumina Infinium Methylation arrays. The Illumina Infinium Human Methylation 450k and MethylationEPIC BeadChip arrays employ two different assays designed to quantify methylation at loci with differing CpG density. (a) The type 1 assay, for CpG-rich intervals, employs two different beads per interrogated CpG position, one for the methylated and unmethylated states following bisulfite conversion. (b) The type II design, for CpG-low regions, uses a single bead type with the methylation state determined following a single base extension after the hybridization step.

Bisulfite NG-Sequencing

There are four common variations on bisulfite sequencing using NGS-technologies, each with different advantages (Table 5.1).

Methyl-seq

Methyl-seq (also known as whole-genome bisulfite sequencing, WGBS; MethylC-seq) theoretically reports the methylation status for the majority of the 28 million CpG sites in the human genome. However, despite being the gold standard for genome-wide methylation analysis, it is extremely expensive, requires a huge bioinformatics effort as at least 1 billion reads of 100 bp end reads are needed to obtain ~30× coverage for each CpG (which equates to four lanes of a HiSeq with 300 million reads each). In this method, genomic DNA is fragmented to which adaptors are ligated, size selected, denatured and treated with sodium bisulfite, with the final libraries generated following PCR amplification. This method determines absolute methylation levels and importantly reveals methylation in sequence context and is only limited by the ability to map unique sequence reads (Table 5.1) (Figure 5.3).

Reduced Representation Bisulfite Sequencing

If the study rational is to assess methylation within CpG-rich sequences then RRBS maybe applicable, allowing for substantial saving on NGS costs, as RRBS libraries typically cover ∼5% of the genome. RRBS utilizes common restriction enzymes that target CpG-rich regions (frequently Msp1) to enrich for small fragments in the 40–220 bp range, which are suitable for sequencing (Table 5.1, Figure 5.3). Because Msp1 is insensitive to methylation and a frequent cutter, the resulting libraries are often biased toward CpG islands and promoters, generally capturing ∼80% of CpG islands and ∼60% of all promoter regions. However, since some promoters have no Msp1 sites these regions will not covered using this method.

Capture-seq

The benefits of high coverage of methyl-seq are hindered by the cost, the necessity for considerable bioinformatic involvement and the large amount of high-quality genomic DNA. Furthermore, methyl-seq has the additional inefficiency that ∼60% of NGS reads provide no methylation information because of they lack CpG sites within the sequence. In addition, bisulfite treatment of DNA effectively doubles the genome size, as both converted (unmethylated) and unconverted (methylated) genome datasets must be collected. Recently, these problems have been addressed with the release of custom DNA-capture kits, tools that selectively enrich CpG containing regions comprehensively and without bias, therefore enabling greater sequence depths, increased sample throughput and lower costs compared to conventions methyl-seq (Table 5.1).

Capture of targeted regions is performed by biotinylated RNA baits that are complementary to target sequences. These probes can be designed to genomic DNA with subsequent bisulfite treatment of the enriched sample (for example, using Agilent's SureSelect Human Methyl-Seq systems) that allow for more than 5.5 million CpGs to be interrogated. Other enrichment protocols allow for the capture of converted DNA where probes target all different possible methylated configurations associated with the regions of interest (as in the case of Roche SeqCap Epi Enrichment) (24). This protocol supports the enrichment of 84 Mb of sequence that contains ∼3.7 million CpG sites. Using standard DNA capture protocols in which bisulfite conversion occurs post-capture requires ∼3 μg of sample to compensate for loss of molecular complexity during library preparation and for damage caused by the harsh bisulfite treatment. However, by performing the bisulfite

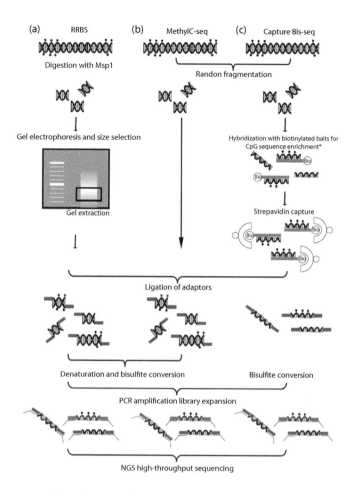

FIGURE 5.3 Genome-wide techniques based on bisulfite conversion. (a) RRBS: Genomic DNA is digested with Msp1 enzyme that recognizes the CCGG motif irrespective of the methylation status of the cytosine. Following digestion, the fragments in the 50–250 bp size range are size-selected, for example by gel extraction, for library preparation and end repair. (b) Methy-seq: Sonicated DNA is directly subject to bisulfite conversion for NGS shotgun sequencing. (c) Captured Bis-seq: This targeted enrichment approach utilizes long biotinylated complementary RNA baits (~120 bp) to capture regions of interest in fragmented DNA samples. Following denaturing and hybridization, the bait: DNA complexes are selected using magnetic streptavidin beads, washed and the RNA baits digested to leave enriched captured DNA for library preparation and downstream applications. For all three techniques the DNA is subject to bisulfite conversion and PCR amplification in which uracils are converted to thymines. The amplification is based on top and bottom strands, which are no longer complementary. For single-end sequencing only the top and bottom strands are sequenced, but for paired-end sequencing all four strands are generated. *Target DNA captured can be before or after bisulfite conversion.

conversion prior to capture, the amount of input can be reduced to 1 μg of sample (Figure 5.3). These protocols are designed to target the same intervals as the HM450k/MethylationEPIC arrays (99% of RefSeq genes) and reveal methylated regions undetected by RRBS and meDIP-seq.

5.3 LOCUS-SPECIFIC METHYLATION ASSESSMENT

It is recognised that targeted approaches are extremely valuable and have been developed to assess methylation at pre-defined loci. For most of these techniques, bisulfite conversion is still required in the initial stages, followed by specific downstream steps. The exception is for methylation-sensitive Multiplex Ligation-dependent Probe Amplification (MS-MLPA) that is widely used in diagnostic labs because it easy to handle and assays are commercially available (Table 5.2).

Bisulfite PCR and Sequencing

Following bisulfite conversion DNA can be used for amplification of the region of interested followed by sequencing of cloned amplicons. Despite being laborious, this technique reveals methylation profiles of each CpG contained within the PCR product, is strand-specific and if the interval contains an informative polymorphism, can give allele-specific information which is essential when studying imprinting. Because the method involves cloning in bacteria, there may be biases against some fragments, leading to errors in methylation state calling. Recently, adaption of this protocol has revealed the existence of strand-specific hemimethylation. Hairpin-bisulfite PCR utilizes a linker that is ligated to Bbvl-cleaved DNA, resulting in attachment of the complementary strands of individual DNA molecules prior to bisulfite conversion and amplification, however, the extent of stable hemimethylation is currently unknown and is likely to be tissue-specific (25). As with most PCR-based technologies there are limitations associated with this method, which applies to all techniques that rely on amplification of converted DNA. Primer design is often problematic due to the reduced complexity of the DNA sequence (although MethPrimer software http://urogene.org/methprimer is recommended) and for unbiased amplification primers should not contain CpG dinucleotides. Frequently, nested PCR is required to overcome non-specific amplification, but the additional rounds of amplification may lead to skews in the population of sequences obtained. Furthermore, amplification of long fragments from a converted DNA is difficult, with an optimal size of 200–350 bp.

Additional Detection Strategies Based on Bisulfite PCR

In addition to cloning of PCR products, several different methods to quantify the methylation, based on the presence of C/T variants have been developed (Table 5.2). These include digesting the resulting PCR amplicons with restriction enzymes that have CG in

TABLE 5.2   Methods for Locus-Specific Methylation Quantification

Method	Description	Advantages	Disadvantages
		Restriction Enzyme-Based Methods	
Southern blot	DNA is digested with methylation-sensitive enzymes and resolved on an agarose gel before transfer to a membrane that is hybridized with a probe.	• Quantitative.	• Laborious. • Requires large quantities of high-molecular weight DNA. • Results only represent the CpGs within the restriction site. • May involve radioactive nucleotide labeling. • Issues of probe specificity.
		Bisulfite Modification-Based Methods	
Cloning and sequencing	Bisulfite-converted DNA is amplified and the products individually cloned in *E.coli* for sequencing.	• Single CpG resolution. • Allele and strand-specific profiles revealed. • Reveals non-CpG methylation.	• Limited to cloning efficiency. • Laborious.
MS-PCR	Bisulfite-modified DNA is amplified with PCR primers designed to target each allele/predicted methylation profile.	• Cheap. • Rapid, ideal for screening.	• Non-quantitative. • Results only represent the CpGs within the primer sequence and not amplicon.
COBRA	Bisulfite-modified DNA is amplified and the resulting PCR products digested with restriction enzymes containing CpG in recognition sequence.	• Cheap. • Rapid, ideal for screening.	• Non-quantitative. • Results only represent the CpGs within the restriction site. • Prone to false-positive/negative results due to incomplete digestion.
MS-SNuPE	Bisulfite-converted DNA is amplified and an internal primer is used for primer extension of cytosine at CpG site.	• Cheap. • Quantitative.	• Requires separate primers for each CpG to be analyzed. • May involve radioactive nucleotide labeling.
Methylight	Bisulfite-converted DNA is amplified and methylation is quantified using fluorescently labeled probes.	• Cheap. • Quantitative.	• Requires separate probes for methylated and unmethylated alleles, which may differ in annealing temperature. • Laborious, required extensive optimization.

(Continued)

TABLE 5.2 (Continued) Methods for Locus-Specific Methylation Quantification

Method	Description	Advantages	Disadvantages
MS-pyrosequencing	Following bisulfite conversion, single stranded PCR products are captured with biotin-tagged primers that are used in sequence reaction. Bioluminometric signal is produced specific to the base incorporated during the extension step by DNA polymerase.	• Quantitative. • Reproducible and fast. • Easy to use. • Allele-specific if the sequencing primer overlaps a heterozygous SNP.	• Limited number of CpG positions analyse due to short sequence length.
Amplicon-seq	Bisulfite-converted DNA is amplified using standard bisulfite PCR and multiple amplicons are simultaneously sequenced using NGS.	• Extremely quantitative. • Single CpG resolution. • Allele & strand-specific profiles revealed. • Reveals non-CpG methylation. • Can accommodate multiplexing of many amplicons in single NGS run.	• Requires basic bioinformatics analysis.
Other Methods			
MassArray	Bisulfite-modified DNA is amplified in multiplex PCR reaction and the products subject to *in vitro* transcription followed by uracil-specific cleavage and mass-spectrometry.	• Commercial and custom assays available. • Semi-quantitative. • Rapid, ideal for screening.	• Unable to discriminate closely positioned CpGs. • Reproducibility issues have been reported. • Does not reveal allele-specific information.
MS-MLPA	MLPA probes are ligated to genomic DNA and the genomic DNA–probe hybrid complexes digested with the Hha1 methylation-sensitive restriction enzyme prior to fluorescent PCR amplification with a single primer pair and capillary electrophoresis.	• Predesigned, optimized assays are commercially available. • Reports both methylation and copy number.	• Not suitable for poor quality/FFPE extracted DNA samples.

their recognition sequence (termed, Combined Bisulfite and Restriction Analysis, COBRA) (26) and high-resolution melt curve analysis (MS-HRM) in which intercalating dye such as SYBRgreen is released upon temperature dissociation. Discrimination of methylated molecules retaining cytosines is based on them having a higher melting temperature compare to unmethylated molecules and would appear as a distinct curve upon dissociation analysis (27).

A more sensitive approach is Methylight, which is based on Taqman® technology, in which methylation is detected by use of methylation-sensitive fluorogenic probes (28) but the gold-standard for locus-specific methylation quantification are pyrosequencing (PyroMark CpG from Qiagen) or deep-bisulfite amplicon sequencing using Roche454 or MiSeq systems (29). Pyrosequencing is based on quantitative SNP calling, with the degree of methylation at each CpG position in a short sequence (up to 100 bp) determined from the ratio of T and C. The process of purification and sequencing can be repeated several times for the same template to analyze other CpGs in the same amplification product (30).

MassARRAY

MassARRAY (commercially offered EpiTYPER assays) starts with bisulfite PCR amplification followed by *in vitro* RNA transcription of the reverse strand, in which C/T variations now appear as G/A that have a mass difference of 16 Da per CpG site that is easily detectable by MALDI-TOF mass spectrometry (31) (Figure 5.4, Table 5.2). The resulting RNA is cleaved by RNAse A and analyzed by mass spectrometry, with distinct and predicable signal patterns resulting for methylated and unmethylated templates. This technique is compatible with multiplexing, as long as the sizes of the predicted cleavage patterns differ, but is unable to analyze multiple closely located CpG positions. Cleavage products containing more than one CpG are termed a "CpG unit" and an average methylation value is assigned. While this is a useful medium-throughput method with a resolution of ~5%, it does suffer from reproducibility issues, which can be limited by increasing experimental replicates, but has been reported to show good correlation with RRBBS data (r > 0.8) (32). Alternatively, by choosing different restriction enzymes, or combinations thereof, it may be possible to tailor the assay to different genomic compartments of interest.

Methylation-Sensitive PCR

This classic technique is useful when large differences in methylation are anticipated, or if imprinted loci are being assessed. Bisulfite PCR is performed with two pairs of primers that are deliberately designed to favor that amplification of methylated or unmethylated DNA molecules by incorporating CpG sequences in the 3′ end of the primer. Staggering of primers and multiplexing methylated/unmethylated pairs results in different-sized amplification products that can be resolved by standard capillary electrophoresis. At best

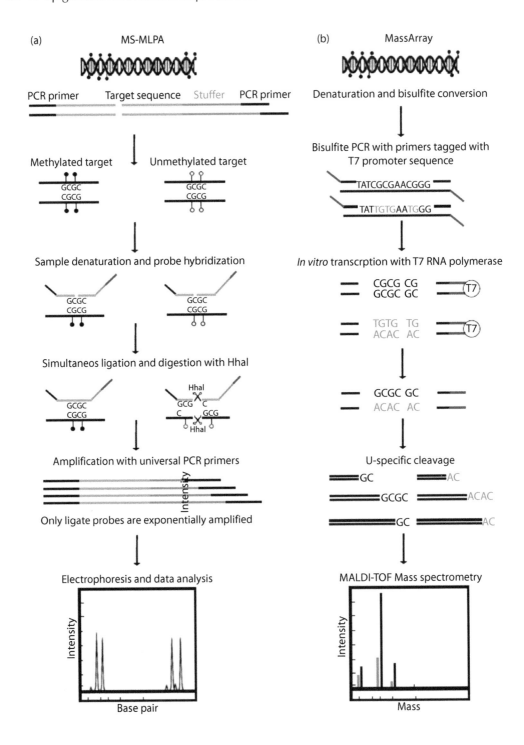

(a) MS-MLPA

(b) MassArray

MS-MLPA (a):

PCR primer | Target sequence | Stuffer | PCR primer

Methylated target | Unmethylated target

GCGC / CGCG

Sample denaturation and probe hybridization

GCGC / CGCG

Simultaneos ligation and digestion with HhaI

HhaI

GCGC / CGCG

Amplification with universal PCR primers

Only ligate probes are exponentially amplified

Electrophoresis and data analysis

Intensity / Base pair

MassArray (b):

Denaturation and bisulfite conversion

Bisulfite PCR with primers tagged with T7 promoter sequence

TATCGCGAACGGG

TATTGTGAATGGG

In vitro transcrption with T7 RNA polymerase

CGCG CG / GCGC GC — T7

TGTG TG / ACAC AC — T7

GCGC GC / ACAC AC

U-specific cleavage

GC / AC

GCGC / ACAC

GC / AC

MALDI-TOF Mass spectrometry

Intensity / Mass

this technique is semi-quantitative, giving information for only the CpGs located under the primers and can be difficult to optimize as methylated and unmethylated oligonucleotides may have different optimal annealing temperatures.

Methylation-Sensitive Multiplex Ligation-Dependent Probe Amplification

MS-MLPA is a multiplex method that measures both methylation and copy-number parameters in a single assay, with many predesigned assays being commercially available (from MRC Holland). This technique relies upon the ligation of MLPA probe oligonucleotides and digestion of the genomic DNA–probe hybrid complexes with the Hha1 methylation-sensitive restriction enzyme prior to fluorescent PCR amplification with a single primer pair. Since each targeted probe contains stuffer sequence of varying length, each interrogated position is visualized as an amplicon of a different size upon capillary electrophoresis (33) (Figure 5.4, Table 5.2).

5.4 METHODS FOR SINGLE-CELL METHYLATION ANALYSIS

Initial Applications Based on NGS Technologies

Almost all methylation profiling methodologies have common limitations: They all require large amounts of starting material, often derived from bulk cell preparations, and have the inherent inability to assess methylation heterogeneity at the individual cell level. To address these issues, low-input and single-cell (sc) bisulfite-based techniques have been developed. Initial advances came from the optimization of the RRBS that integrated the Mspl digestion step with the bisulfite conversion within a single tube. This provided methylation

---

FIGURE 5.4   Commercially available techniques for low-throughput methylation analyses. (a) MS-MLPA: Both the copy number and methylation of the target DNA is simultaneously assessed with this technique using multiple methylation-sensitive probes. The probes are designed to sequences that contain a methylation-sensitive Hha1 restriction site (GCGC). After probe hybridization, the reaction is split into two equal parts, one for the copy number, the other for methylation profiling following Hha1 digestion. When the probe encounters non-methylated target sequences, the probes will be ligated and simultaneously digested with Hha1, destroying the template for subsequent PCR amplification. However, if the target sequence is methylated the Hha1 site will be refractory to digestion and amplification can occur resulting in a peak signal following electrophoresis. (b) MassArray: This method starts with bisulfite conversion of the genomic DNA, followed by PCR amplification using primers that are tagged with the T7-promoter sequence. Next, *in vitro* transcription is performed on the reverse strand, followed by base-specific cleavage using RNaseA at specific U or C bases. MALD-TOF MS analysis of the cleavage products reveals specific patterns, the sizes of which can be predicted for methylated and unmethylated molecules.

information for approximately 1 million CpG sites, and has been instrumental in profiling the dynamics of embryonic reprograming following fertilization (34–36). To overcome PCR-induced duplicated read bias that may occur during low-input and scRRBS library preparation, unique molecule identifiers (UMIs) can be incorporated during the library preparations. This has been shown to successfully allow accurate quantification of DNA molecules and to reveal allele-specific methylation patterns (37). However RRBS cannot be used to examine all regions of interest unless the appropriate restriction enzyme sites adequately flank them. Subsequently, an adaption of the methyl-seq protocol, namely Post-Bisulfite Adaptor Tagging sequencing (PBAT-seq), has increased genome coverage by taking advantage of one of the drawbacks of bisulfite treatment, the spontaneous fragmentation of DNA template that results from the chemical reaction (38). By performing bisulfite conversion before adaptor tagging, the DNA is fragmented by the treatment itself, resulting in the ability to use lower amounts of starting material. PBAT-seq is now applicable to single cells, with reports of coverage of >50% of CpG sites and by combining data from a few as 20 individual cells, has allowed for the whole methylome of mouse oocytes to be determined (39). Furthermore, the scPBAT-seq protocol is also compatible with automated liquid-handling robots, which allows for the processing of a large number of cells with increases in success rates and the proportion of informative sequences in a time-efficient manner (40).

Single-Cell Multi-Omics Protocols

Single-cell sequencing technologies have greatly helped dissect the heterogeneity of different cells present within a sample. In addition to scPBAT-seq and scRRBS, single-cell epigenome methods such as scHi-Seq, scChIP-seq, scDNAsel-seq, and scATAC-seq have revealed the wider epigenetic and chromatin heterogeneity in cell populations (41). All of these methods currently suffer from problems of spare coverage and poor signal-to-noise ratios. The simultaneous measurement of different layers of epigenetic information from the same cell remains challenging. One multi-omics protocol, Chromatin Overall Omics-scale Landscape sequencing (COOL-seq) allows for the assessment of chromatin accessibility, nucleosome positioning and DNA methylation (42). This method is essentially a scaled-down combination of Nucleosome Occupancy and Methylome sequencing (NOMe-seq), by which accessible chromatin is probes by sensitivity to methylation by the bacterial M.CviP1 methyltransferase, and scPBAT-seq, which has been shown to be sensitive and robust at the single-cell level.

Adaption of the recently described genome and transcriptome sequencing (G&T-seq) protocol (43), which allows for the physical separation of polyadenylated mRNA from genomic DNA, has been used to simultaneously profile expression and methylation in individual cells. This technology, termed M&T-seq, adds a bisulfite conversion step following genomic DNA isolation, allowing for the direct correlation between methylation and transcriptome dynamics at single-cell resolution (44). M&T-se has been successfully combined with NOME-seq to enable the parallel analysis of DNA methylation, gene expression and chromatin accessibility within single cells. Although there is some loss of CpG methylation data implicit in the assay, the mean per cell coverage of accessibility at promoter elements is very high at ~70% (45).

Low-Input and Single-Cell Locus-Specific Assays

As with all NGS-based techniques that are primarily used as discovery platforms, the next step is to validate the results using locus-specific methods. Several locus-specific methods have been modified for low-input and single-cell methylation confirmation and in each case technical artefacts, such as PCR amplification bias, have to be rigorously controlled.

One of the first techniques developed was designed to specifically exploit methylation-sensitive restriction enzymes in an approach based called SCRAM, and this method was successfully used to reveal epigenetic chimerisim and imprinting dynamics in early mouse embryos (46). Essentially, SCRAM combines single-cell MSRE digestions with multiplexed PCR analysis in which DNA is digested with a restriction enzyme that only cleaves DNA if the specific recognition sequence is unmethylated (Figure 5.5, Table 5.3). All the target loci of interest are simultaneously co-amplified with a limited-cycle multiplexed pre-amplification PCR using two forward primers and a reverse primer for each locus. The two forward primers are designed to flank the recognition site, such that two PCR products (one long product including the restriction site and one short product excluding the restriction site) can be obtained with a single reverse primer. If the sample template DNA was methylated and undigested, both products can be amplified, whereas only the short PCR product is obtained if the initial template DNA was unmethylated and thus cleaved. Subsequently the pre-amplification product is divided into individual reaction for target-specific amplification to determine whether the original site is methylated (both the long and short fragments are detectable by qPCR) or unmethylated (only the short fragment is detectable by qPCR). This method has important advantages in that it controls for degradation of single-copy genomic DNA that could manifest itself as allele dropout and scalability, having recently been adapted for use with a Fluidigm microfluidic-multiplexed qPCR chip (47).

A second low-input locus-specific assay has recently been used to describe imprinting profiles in single human embryos based on nested-multiple bisulfite PCR. This method relies on the ability to directly denature and convert DNA in cell lysates cells using sodium bisulfite in a single step (using the EZ DNA methylation-Direct Kit). The recovered bisulfite-converted DNA is then used in a first round multiplexed bisulfite PCR in which multiple loci are co-amplified, followed by individual locus-specific nested PCR reactions on an aliquot of the first reaction (48) (Figure 5.5, Table 5.3). Although this technique requiring high cycles

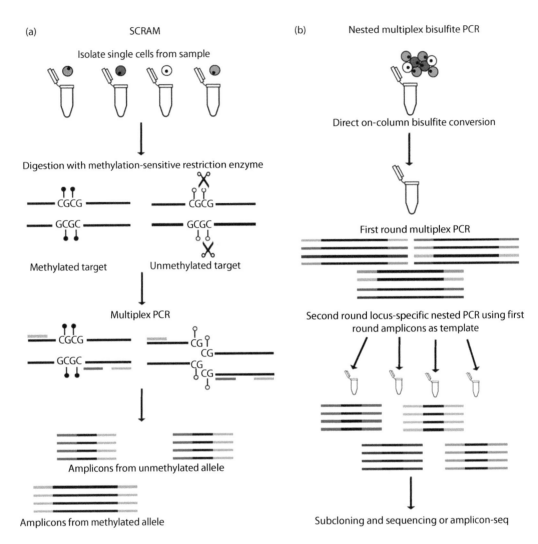

FIGURE 5.5 Locus-specific techniques for methylation profiling of single-cell/low-input samples. (a) SCRAM: Cellular DNA is digested with the restriction enzyme BstU1 (CGCG) for which methylation prevents cleavage. Subsequently, a multiplex PCR reaction is performed using two different "forward primers" located on either side of the BstU1 site, utilizing a common "reverse primer." If the DNA is methylated, both primer combinations will generate PCR products subtly differing in size. However, if the DNA is unmethylated and cut with BstU1, the larger amplicon cannot be generated. (b) Nested-multiplex bisulfite PCR: During the first round of PCR reactions all "outer" primers are co-amplified in a multiplex reaction. This product is subsequently split into equal fractions for second round of amplifications using locus-specific "inner" nested primers. Following confirmation of specific amplification by gel electrophoresis, the PCR products are purified and cloned into *E. coli* and individual clones are sequenced.

TABLE 5.3   Methods for Single-Cell/Low-Input Methylation Quantification

Method	Description	Advantages	Disadvantages
SCRAM	Single-cell methylation-sensitive restriction enzyme digestion with multiplexed PCR analysis in which primers are designed to flank the recognition sites, therefore discriminating methylation based on the ability to amplify undigested/methylated DNA.	• Ideal for single-cell and low-input samples. • Builtin controls for digestion. • Scalable, can be used in multiplexed qPCR, up to 24 loci per cell. • Adaptable to microfluidic platforms.	• Reactions may fail/false results obtained due to incomplete digestion. • Assays limited to CpGs in methylation-sensitive restriction enzyme sites. • No allele-specific information. • Assumption that single CpG site per region is representative of methylation status of the locus of interest.
Nested multiplex Bis-PCR	Bisulfite-converted DNA is subject to two rounds of amplification. The first is multiplexed, the product of which is used as a template for the second PCR utilizing locus-specific internal nested primers.	• Scalable, >20 loci can be analyzed in a single sample. • Single CpG resolution. • Allele and strand-specific profiles revealed. • Compatible with cloning and sequencing or amplicon-seq.	• Laborious, required extensive optimization to avoid amplification bias. • All bisulfite PCRs must have similar efficiencies and annealing temperatures. • Requires bisulfite conversion, inefficient for single-cell use.
scBS-seq/scPBAT-seq	A single-tube reaction strategy based on bisulfite conversion followed by random priming and adaptor incorporation for library generation.	• Approximately 3.5 million CpG sites can be assessed in each cell. • Sequences include both CpG islands and CpG-sparse regions.	• Due to the random nature of the sequences obtained, there may be limited overlap between individual cells making comparison of specific loci between cells difficult. • Loss of strand information because of repeat rounds of random priming. • Requires extensive bioinformatic analysis.
scRRBS	Standard RRBS optimized for single cells with modified volumes and single-tube reactions for purification, digestion, end repair and dA tailing, adaptor ligation, and bisulfite conversion to avoid unnecessary DNA loss.	• Approximately 2 million CpG sites can be assessed in each cell, mainly mapping to CpG islands.	• Single-tube approach may affect coverage compared to standard RRBS. • Owing to bisulfite degradation of DNA, both alleles are very rarely sequenced at a given locus. • Requires extensive bioinformatic analysis.

of amplification, careful primer design limits PCR bias. In addition, since the methylation profiles of the final PCR products are determined by subcloning and Sanger sequencing, methylation information for multiple CpGs is reported, as are allelic-specific profiles if heterozygous single nucleotide sequence variants are present in the final amplicons.

5.5 PROTOCOLS FOR DETECTING 5hmC

Studies in recent years have revealed that 5hmC is present in many tissues (49,50). The TET enzymes are responsible for converting 5mC to 5hmC through Fe(II)/α-ketoglutarate-dependent hydroxylation (6). However, it is unclear whether 5hmC is simply an intermediate of the DNA demethylation process, or if it possesses its own singular epigenetic function. The detection of 5hmC is technically more challenging than 5mC due to the low abundance of 5hmC and because bisulfite treatment cannot distinguish between the two forms because 5hmC is also resistant to deamination, so that analyses on classic bisulfite-converted DNA will provide combined data for 5mC plus 5hmC (17). One of the first methods to address the quantification of 5hmC was a modified protocol of meDIP that utilized a highly specific anti-5hmC antibody (hmeDIP), for which the immunoselected DNA molecules could be used for subsequent PCR or NGS interrogation (51).

More recently, modifications to the standard bisulfite conversion (for example the TrueMethyl kit from CEGX), which incorporate a highly selective oxidation step, have become popular. The oxidative bisulfite (oxBS) treatment of DNA allows for discrimination between 5mC and 5hmC via selective chemical oxidation of 5hmC to 5fC (52). The latter derivative deaminates to uracil during bisulfite treatment, so that the only cytosine base not deaminated following oxBS is 5mC. Several publications have demonstrated that oxBS conversion can be incorporated into both the NGS-technologies and Illumina Infinium BeadChip array protocols to facilitate the genome-wide quantification of both 5mC and 5hmC (53). Subtraction of oxBS-generated methylation from standard bisulfite profiles allows for the detection of 5hmC at cytosine positions throughout the genome. An important consideration is that very deeply sequenced data are required to infer locus-specific 5hmC levels accurately. This approach has been used to characterize the 5hmC patterns in different tissues, revealing that 5hmC is substantially enriched in the brain compared with leukocytes (54) and the placenta (55), observations that confirm initial reports using both mass spectrometry and antibody-based technologies (56).

The resulting DNA from either hmeDIP and oxBS treatment can we used for locus-specific PCR confirmation. An additional confirmation method that discriminates 5mC from 5hmC is the T4 ß-glucosyltransferase (T4-BGT) assay (57). This method distinguishes the two methylated forms by the addition of a glucose-moiety to the hydroxyl group of 5hmC that results in non-cleavable Msp1 sites which subsequently act as template for qPCR.

Alternative methods for detecting the genome-wide 5hmC distribution patterns have recently been described which complement the approaches described above. The use of a unique DNA-modification-dependent restriction endonuclease AbaSI (58) coupled with sequencing (Aba-seq) reveals the precise location of 5hmC when cleaved ends are mapped. Results using this technique confirm that 5hmC is relatively abundant in intergenic regions and closely mirrors the 5mC profile, is depleted in CpG islands, with non-CG hydroxymethylation prevalent in the mitochondrial genome (59). A similar genome-wide distribution was also observed using a different technique with single-base 5hmC resolution. TET-assisted bisulfite sequencing (TAB-seq) utilizes T4-BGT-mediated protection of 5hmC with TET1-based oxidation of 5mC allowing for the distinction of 5hmC from unmodified cytosine and 5mC by genome-wide or locus-specific sequencing (60).

5.6 THIRD-GENERATION SEQUENCING

One of the main limitations of the NGS-based bisulfite techniques is the short read lengths, which hamper sequence read mappability and only give short-range contiguous methylation patterns. Two different third-generation sequence technologies, Pacific Biosciences PACBIO single-molecule real-time (SMRT) sequencing and Nanopore sequencing allow for the quantification of unmodified bases, not only restricted to cytosines (including N6-methyladenine and N4-methylcytosine) (Figure 5.6). The PACBIO RSII instrument directly detects 5mC, 5hmC, and unmodified bases in untreated DNA by analyzing polymerase kinetics in long sequence reads, which have been reported to average ~3 kb (61). In addition, 5mC can also be detected in differential electric current signals measured on Nanopore-based sequence devices. Recently, 5mC was characterized using the Oxford Nanopore Technologies MinION instrument (62) with a reported resolution of ~10 bp between individual CpG sites for 3.5–6 kb fragments. Although the detection of modified bases using these technologies offer huge promise, these techniques require considerable optimization and bioinformatics processing before they can be considered established techniques since they are limited by the high error rate, high costs and the requirement for a large amount of native, unamplified DNA template.

5.7 CONCLUDING REMARKS

This chapter provides an overview of the current technologies for the assessment of DNA methylation, with simple descriptions while highlighting advantages and disadvantages of each method. Readers can also select the most appropriate techniques for the biological samples to be studied and which method best addresses their research question. For example, in relation to reproductive epigenetics, if genomic DNA is not a limiting factor, for example in the profiling of DNA derived from patient blood, placenta biopsies, or bulk sperm samples, then genome-wide multiple comparisons can be performed using high-density methylation

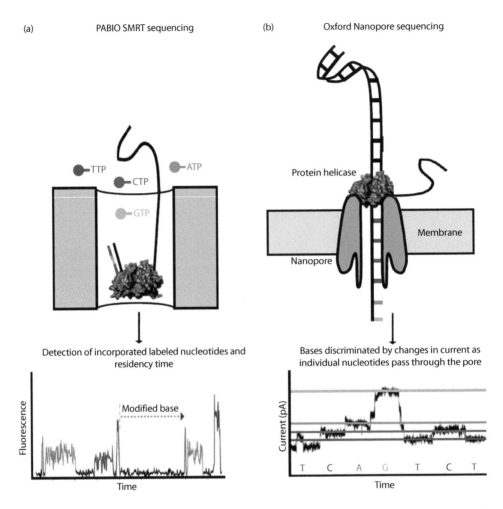

(a) PABIO SMRT sequencing   (b) Oxford Nanopore sequencing

FIGURE 5.6 Third-generation methylation profiling. (a) SMRT sequencing. A single immobilized polymerase molecule is attached to the bottom of a well, called a zero-mode waveguide (ZMW), thousands of which make up a SMRT cell. Each of the four fluorescent-labeled nucleotides is added to the SMRT cell and as bases associate with the polymerase, a specific light pulse is produced that identifies the base. The replication processes in all ZMWs of a SMRT cell are recorded as a "movie" of light pulses, which are subsequently interpreted as a DNA sequence. Alterations in the predicted rates of incorporation dictate a modified base. (b) Nanopore sequencing. An enzyme ratchet unwinds double-stranded DNA so that single-stranded molecules can pass through a protein nanopore. An ionic current trace is altered in the surrounding membrane when the DNA molecule is passing through the nanopore, with each nucleotide, and their modifications, resulting in a characteristic disruption in current potential. These current changes are then decoded to give a DNA sequence in real time. Since this technique generates data irrespective of length of the DNA molecules, hard to sequence loci, such as repeats, can be assessed.

arrays or targeted methyl-seq, followed by confirmation with quantitative locus-specific assays. This strategy has been used to decipher the mechanisms associated with IUGR (63), pre-eclampsia (64–66), endometrial responsiveness (67,68), male factor infertility (69–71), and to study epigenetic stability following assisted reproductive techniques (72).

If the quantities of DNA are limiting, which is often the case when studying embryos or oocytes, then single-cell or protocols optimized for low input samples will reveal sample heterogeneity while given high-genome coverage. In these cases, sequence depth is important, as samples with low coverage will be associated with high false-discovery rates following bioinformatic analysis.

Furthermore, methylation profiling has recently been used to identify circulating cell-free fetal DNA in maternal circulation as a means of non-invasive diagnosis of chromosomal abnormalities (73). Overall, the ongoing advances in technology with the implementation of low-input and single-cell applications will allow for the development of precise and affordable methods for embryo selection and accurate monitoring of gamete quality.

REFERENCES

1. Okano M, Bell DW, Haber DA, Li E. DNA methyltransferases Dnmt3a and Dnmt3b are essential for *de novo* methylation and mammalian development. *Cell*. 1999;99:247–57.
2. Barau J, Teissandier A, Zamudio N et al. The DNA methyltransferase DNMT3C protects male germ cells from transposon activity. *Science*. 2016;354:909–12.
3. Li E, Bestor TH, Jaenisch R. Targeted mutation of the DNA methyltransferase gene results in embryonic lethality. *Cell*. 1992;69:915–26.
4. Monk D. Germline-derived DNA methylation and early embryo epigenetic reprogramming: The selected survival of imprints. *Int J Biochem Cell Biol*. 2015;67:128–38.
5. Heyn H, Esteller M. An adenine code for DNA: A second life for N6-methyladenine. *Cell*. 2015;161:710–3.
6. Tahiliani M, Koh KP, Shen Y et al. Conversion of 5-methylcytosine to 5-hydroxymethylcytosine in mammalian DNA by MLL partner TET1. *Science*. 2009;324:930–5.
7. de Koning AP, Gu W, Castoe TA et al. Repetitive elements may comprise over two-thirds of the human genome. *PLoS Genet*. 2011;7:e1002384.
8. Du Q, Luu PL, Stirzaker C, Clark SJ. Methyl-CpG-binding domain proteins: Readers of the epigenome. *Epigenomics*. 2015;7:1051–73.
9. Thomson JP, Skene PJ, Selfridge J et al. CpG islands influence chromatin structure via the CpG-binding protein Cfp1. *Nature*. 2010;464:1082–6.
10. Sharp AJ, Stathaki E, Migliavacca E et al. DNA methylation profiles of human active and inactive X chromosomes. *Genome Res*. 2011;21:1592–600.
11. Gahurova L, Tomizawa SI, Smallwood SA et al. Transcription and chromatin determinants of *de novo* DNA methylation timing in oocytes. *Epigenetics Chromatin*. 2017;10:25.
12. Kuo KC, McCune RA, Gehrke CW et al. Quantitative reversed-phase high performance liquid chromatographic determination of major and modified deoxyribonucleosides in DNA. *Nucleic Acids Res*. 1980;8:4763–76.

13. Le T, Kim KP, Fan G, Faull KF. A sensitive mass spectrometry method for simultaneous quantification of DNA methylation and hydroxymethylation levels in biological samples. *Anal Biochem*. 2011;412:203–9.

14. Cedar H, Solage A, Glaser G, Razin A. Direct detection of methylated cytosine in DNA by use of the restriction enzyme MspI. *Nucleic Acids Res*. 1979;6:2125–32.

15. Hatada I, Sugama T, Mukai T. A new imprinted gene cloned by a methylation-sensitive genome scanning method. *Nucleic Acids Res*. 1993;21:5577–82.

16. Kelsey G, Bodle D, Miller HJ et al. Identification of imprinted loci by methylation-sensitive representational difference analysis: Application to mouse distal chromosome 2. *Genomics*. 1999;62:129–38.

17. Frommer M, McDonald LE, Millar DS et al. A genomic sequencing protocol that yields a positive display of 5-methylcytosine residues in individual DNA strands. *Proc Natl Acad Sci USA*. 1992;89:1827–31.

18. Bock C, Tomazou EM, Brinkman AB et al. Quantitative comparison of genome-wide DNA methylation mapping technologies. *Nat Biotechnol*. 2010;28:1106–14.

19. Harris RA, Wang T, Coarfa C et al. Comparison of sequencing-based methods to profile DNA methylation and identification of monoallelic epigenetic modifications. *Nat Biotechnol*. 2010;28:1097–105.

20. Rauch T, Pfeifer GP. Methylated-CpG island recovery assay: A new technique for the rapid detection of methylated-CpG islands in cancer. *Lab Invest*. 2005;85:1172–80.

21. Moran S, Arribas C, Esteller M. Validation of a DNA methylation microarray for 850,000 CpG sites of the human genome enriched in enhancer sequences. *Epigenomics*. 2016;8:389–99.

22. Bibikova M, Barnes B, Tsan C et al. High density DNA methylation array with single CpG site resolution. *Genomics*. 2011;98:288–95.

23. Court F, Tayama C, Romanelli V et al. Genome-wide parent-of-origin DNA methylation analysis reveals the intricacies of human imprinting and suggests a germline methylation-independent mechanism of establishment. *Genome Res*. 2014;24:554–69.

24. Li Q, Suzuki M, Wendt J et al. Post-conversion targeted capture of modified cytosines in mammalian and plant genomes. *Nucleic Acids Res*. 2015;43:e81.

25. Patiño-Parrado I, Gómez-Jiménez Á, López-Sánchez N, Frade JM. Strand-specific CpG hemimethylation, a novel epigenetic modification functional for genomic imprinting. *Nucleic Acids Res*. 2017;45:8822–34.

26. Xiong Z, Laird PW. COBRA: A sensitive and quantitative DNA methylation assay. *Nucleic Acids Res*. 1997;25:2532–4.

27. Wojdacz TK, Dobrovic A. Methylation-sensitive high resolution melting (MS-HRM): A new approach for sensitive and high-throughput assessment of methylation. *Nucleic Acids Res*. 2007;35:e41.

28. Eads CA, Danenberg KD, Kawakami K et al. MethyLight: A high-throughput assay to measure DNA methylation. *Nucleic Acids Res*. 2000;28:E32.

29. Beygo J, Ammerpohl O, Gritzan D et al. Deep bisulphite sequencing of aberrantly methylated loci in a patient with multiple methylation defects. *PLoS One*. 2013;8:e76953.

30. Tost J, Gut IG. DNA methylation analysis by pyrosequencing. *Nat Protoc*. 2007;2:2265–75.

31. Ehrich M, Nelson MR, Stanssens P et al. Quantitative high-throughput analysis of DNA methylation patterns by base-specific cleavage and mass spectrometry. *Proc Natl Acad Sci USA*. 2005;102:15785–90.

32. Chatterjee A, Macaulay EC, Ahn A et al. Comparative assessment of DNA methylation patterns between reduced representation bisulphite sequencing and Sequenom EpiTyper methylation analysis. *Epigenomics.* 2017;9:823–32.
33. Priolo M, Sparago A, Mammi C et al. MS-MLPA is a specific and sensitive technique for detecting all chromosome 11p15.5 imprinting defects of BWS and SRS in a single-tube experiment. *E J Hum Genet.* 2008;16:565–71.
34. Smallwood SA, Tomizawa S, Krueger F et al. Dynamic CpG island methylation landscape in oocytes and preimplantation embryos. *Nat Genet.* 2011;43:811–4.
35. Guo H, Zhu P, Yan L et al. The DNA methylation landscape of human early embryos. *Nature.* 2014;511:606–10.
36. Smith ZD, Chan MM, Humm KC et al. DNA methylation dynamics of the human preimplantation embryo. *Nature.* 2014;511:611–5.
37. Wang K, Li X, Dong S et al. Q-RRBS: A quantitative reduced representation bisulphite sequencing method for single-cell methylome analyses. *Epigenetics.* 2015;10:775–83.
38. Miura F, Ito T. Highly sensitive targeted methylome sequencing by post-bisulphite adaptor tagging. *DNA Res.* 2015;22:13–8.
39. Smallwood SA, Lee HJ, Angermueller C et al. Single-cell genome-wide bisulphite sequencing for assessing epigenetic heterogeneity. *Nat Methods.* 2014;11:817–20.
40. Clark SJ, Lee HJ, Smallwood SA et al. Single-cell epigenomics: Powerful new methods for understanding gene regulation and cell identity. *Genome Biol.* 2016;17:72.
41. Kelsey G, Stegle O, Reik W. Single-cell epigenomics: Recording the past and predicting the future. *Science.* 2017;358:69–75.
42. Guo F, Li L, Li J et al. Single-cell multi-omics sequencing of mouse early embryos and embryonic stem cells. *Cell Res.* 2017;27:967–88.
43. Macaulay IC, Teng MJ, Haerty W et al. Separation and parallel sequencing of the genomes and transcriptomes of single cells using G&T-seq. *Nat Protoc.* 2016;11:2081–103.
44. Angermueller C, Clark SJ, Lee HJ et al. Parallel single-cell sequencing links transcriptional and epigenetic heterogeneity. *Nat Methods.* 2016;13:229–32.
45. Lorthongpanich C, Cheow LF, Balu S et al. Single-cell DNA-methylation analysis reveals epigenetic chimerism in preimplantation embryos. *Science.* 2013;341:1110–2.
46. Clark SJ, Argelaguet R, Kapourani CA et al. scNMT-seq enables joint profiling of chromatin accessibility DNA methylation and transcription in single cells. *BioRxiv.* 2017. doi: https://doi.org/10.1101/138685.
47. Cheow LF, Quake SR, Burkholder WF, Messerschmidt DM. Multiplexed locus-specific analysis of DNA methylation in single cells. *Nat Protoc.* 2015;10:619–31.
48. Sanchez-Delgado M, Court F, Vidal E et al. Human oocyte-derived methylation differences persist in the placenta revealing widespread transient imprinting. *PLoS Genet.* 2016;12:e1006427.
49. Globisch D, Münzel M, Müller M et al. Tissue distribution of 5-hydroxymethylcytosine and search for active demethylation intermediates. *PLoS One.* 2010;5:e15367.
50. Nestor CE, Ottaviano R, Reddington J et al. Tissue type is a major modifier of the 5-hydroxymethylcytosine content of human genes. *Genome Res.* 2012;22:467–77.
51. Nestor CE, Meehan RR. Hydroxymethylated DNA immunoprecipitation (hmeDIP). *Methods Mol Biol.* 2014;1094:259–67.

52. Booth MJ, Marsico G, Bachman M et al. Quantitative sequencing of 5-formylcytosine in DNA at single-base resolution. *Nat Chem.* 2014;6:435–40.

53. Lunnon K, Hannon E, Smith RG et al. Variation in 5-hydroxymethylcytosine across human cortex and cerebellum. *Genome Biol.* 2016;17:27.

54. Stewart SK, Morris TJ, Guilhamon P et al. oxBS-450K: A method for analysing hydroxymethylation using 450 K BeadChips. *Methods.* 2015;72:9–15.

55. Hernandez Mora JR, Sanchez-Delgado M, Petazzi P et al. Profiling of oxBS-450 K 5-hydroxymethylcytosine in human placenta and brain reveals enrichment at imprinted loci. *Epigenetics.* 2017 [Epub ahead of print]

56. Globisch D, Münzel M, Müller M et al. Tissue distribution of 5-hydroxymethylcytosine and search for active demethylation intermediates. *PLoS One.* 2010;5:e15367.

57. Song CX, Szulwach KE, Fu Y et al. Selective chemical labeling reveals the genome-wide distribution of 5-hydroxymethylcytosine. *Nat Biotechnol.* 2011;29:68–72.

58. Wang H, Guan S, Quimby A et al. Comparative characterization of the PvuRts1I family of restriction enzymes and their application in mapping genomic 5-hydroxymethylcytosine. *Nucleic Acids Res.* 2011;39:9294–305.

59. Sun Z, Terragni J, Borgaro J et al. High-resolution enzymatic mapping of genomic 5-hydroxymethylcytosine in mouse embryonic stem cells. *Cell Reports.* 2013;3:567–76.

60. Yu M, Hons G, Szulwach K et al. Base-Resolution Analysis of 5-Hydroxymethylcytosine in the Mammalian Genome. *Cell.* 2012;149:1368–80.

61. Beaulaurier J, Zhang XS, Zhu S et al. Single molecule-level detection and long read-based phasing of epigenetic variations in bacterial methylomes. *Nat Commun.* 2015;6:7438.

62. Simpson JT, Workman RE, Zuzarte PC et al. Detecting DNA cytosine methylation using nanopore sequencing. *Nat Methods.* 2017;14:407–10.

63. Hillman SL, Finer S, Smart MC et al. Novel DNA methylation profiles associated with key gene regulation and transcription pathways in blood and placenta of growth-restricted neonates. *Epigenetics.* 2015;10:50–61.

64. Anton L, Brown AG, Bartolomei MS, Elovitz MA. Differential methylation of genes associated with cell adhesion in preeclamptic placentas. *PLoS One.* 2014;9:e100148.

65. Chu T, Bunce K, Shaw P et al. Comprehensive analysis of preeclampsia-associated DNA methylation in the placenta. *PLoS One.* 2014;9:e107318.

66. Zhu L, Lv R, Kong L et al. Genome-wide mapping of 5mC and 5hmC identified differentially modified genomic regions in late-onset severe preeclampsia: A pilot study. *PLoS One.* 2015;10:e0134119.

67. Saare M, Modhukur V, Suhorutshenko M et al. The influence of menstrual cycle and endometriosis on endometrial methylome. *Clin Epigenetics.* 2016;8:2.

68. Kukushkina V, Modhukur V, Suhorutšenko M et al. DNA methylation changes in endometrium and correlation with gene expression during the transition from pre-receptive to receptive phase. *Sci Rep.* 2017;7:3916.

69. Hammoud SS, Nix DA, Zhang H et al. Distinctive chromatin in human sperm packages genes for embryo development. *Nature.* 2009;460:473–8.

70. Schütte B, El Hajj N, Kuhtz J et al. Broad DNA methylation changes of spermatogenesis, inflammation and immune response-related genes in a subgroup of sperm samples for assisted reproduction. *Andrology.* 2013;1:822–9.

71. Camprubí C, Salas-Huetos A, Aiese-Cigliano R et al. Spermatozoa from infertile patients exhibit differences of DNA methylation associated with spermatogenesis-related processes: An array-based analysis. *Reprod Biomed Online.* 2016;33:709–19.

72. Camprubí C, Iglesias-Platas I, Martin-Trujillo A et al. Stability of genomic imprinting and gestational-age dynamic methylation in complicated pregnancies conceived following assisted reproductive technologies. *Biol Reprod.* 2013;89:50.

73. Nygren AO, Dean J, Jensen TJ et al. Quantification of fetal DNA by use of methylation-based DNA discrimination. *Clin Chem.* 2010;56:1627–35.

CHAPTER 6

Intrinsic and Extrinsic Factors That Influence Epigenetics

Ivan Nalvarte, Joëlle Rüegg, and Carlos Guerrero-Bosagna

CONTENTS

6.1 INTRODUCTION

The original definition of *Epigenetics* by Conrad Waddington was "The branch of biology which studies the causal interactions between genes and their products which bring phenotypes into being" (1). As can be seen, this original definition is already aimed at describing how factors involved in the development of organisms (i.e., the "epi" part of epigenetics) affect the expression of their genetic composition.

Nowadays, the focus of epigenetics has shifted to study accessory chemical modifications on the DNA that are able to regulate gene expression and survive mitotic events (2). However, epigenetic mechanisms still represent processes that bridge the gap between environmental influences and long-term regulation of gene expression, which is in turn involved in phenotype formation.

Every epigenetic process described to date has two basic components: The intrinsic machinery of the cells and the contribution of external factors. External factors will act on the epigenetic machineries by: (i) providing chemicals as substrate for the epigenetic reactions, (ii) affecting the functioning of enzymes that are involved in epigenetic reactions, or (iii) altering the binding of ligands to receptors that respond to environmental stimuli, and that subsequently trigger cascade of reactions that will ultimately affect the epigenetic machinery.

Epigenetic machineries are involved in any aspect of the body's function. In the following sections we will describe the role of intrinsic (endogenous) factors in influencing epigenetic regulation related to reproductive health, followed by a description of extrinsic (environmentally available) factors that, in one way or another, alter the functioning of epigenetic machineries in the developing and adult organism and thereby may affect its reproductive capacity. First, however, we provide some basic information about epigenetic mechanisms and processes.

6.2 DEVELOPMENTAL PERIODS OF EPIGENETIC REPROGRAMMING

At the interface of the interaction between intrinsic and extrinsic factors are developmental periods of "epigenetic reprogramming". Special susceptibility for the action of environmental compounds occurs during these periods that involve transient albeit major epigenetic rearrangements. Two waves of extensive epigenetic reprogramming are described to date in mammals. One is after fertilization, where an initial reduction in DNA methylation is followed by re-methylation at the time of blastocyst implantation (3). This epigenetic reprogramming is crucial for the differentiation of somatic cells. Another period of epigenetic reprogramming occurs during the migration of primordial germ cells (PGCs) toward their final establishment in the gonads (4). During this migration a major demethylation of the genome also occurs followed by re-methylation (3–5). This epigenetic reprogramming is crucial for the differentiation of somatic cells.

Disruptions in epigenetic reprograming triggered by environmental factors have different consequences depending on whether blastocysts or germ cells are affected. When environmental exposures (such as endocrine disruptors) affect preimplantation embryos, important somatic phenotypic and epigenetic effects will be produced in the individuals emerging from these embryos (6,7). However, when the epigenetic reprogramming of primordial germ cells is affected, the epigenetic disruption could affect individuals in the next generations (8–10). Although in the following generations epigenetic reprogramming will also occur, thereby erasing most of the epigenetic marks brought from previous generations, epigenetic marks will persist in genomic regions known as "escapees" (11). Such regions could be responsible for the transgenerational transmission of phenotypic effects induced by environmental insults.

6.3 INTRINSIC FACTORS INFLUENCING EPIGENETIC PROCESSES AND REGULATING REPRODUCTIVE HEALTH

Many endogenous factors shown to alter epigenetic mechanisms relate to the endocrine system, which have distinct roles at different ontogenetic stages. Due to this, we have separated the description of the endogenous factors on epigenetic systems according to different developmental and reproductive stages: Pre- and early postnatal development, puberty, and adulthood.

Pre- and Early Postnatal Development

The development of fetal germ cells is mediated by the release of luteinizing hormone (LH) and follicle stimulating hormone (FSH) from the fetal gonadotrope-precursor cells (GnPCs) located at the developing anterior pituitary. Studies in mouse models have shown that germ cell proliferation and differentiation is similar in both sexes until 10.5 days post coitum (dpc). Thereafter, germ cell development starts to become sex-specific (12).

Embryonic LH production appears to be under intricate epigenetic control. It has recently been shown that expression of the *Lh* gene in mice is orchestrated by the active DNA demethylation involving Tet1 and Tet2 enzymes (13). Interestingly, mice lacking Tet1/2 are viable but show abnormal ovarian development and reduced fertility (14) pointing toward an important role of Tet enzymes in ovarian development. In addition, the regulation of Tet1 expression and activity in differentiating GnPCs is regulated by liganded estrogen and androgen receptors, and the gonadotropin-releasing hormone (GnRH) through activation of protein kinase A (PKA) (13), suggesting that proper hormonal signaling is decisive in the epigenetic control of ovarian development.

A key factor responsible for the initiation of male sexual differentiation is the Y-chromosome encoded transcription factor SRY (sex-determining on the Y chromosome), which controls the expression of different genes involved in male gonadal development and thus the increase in perinatal testosterone levels (15,16). In the developing mouse testes, DNA demethylation of a regulatory region of the *Sry* gene occurs at 11.5 dpc and correlates with increased expression of *Sry* (17). This demethylation is testis specific and is believed to be mediated by GADD45 (growth arrest DNA damage-inducible 45) proteins that recruit DNA repair proteins to replace methylated cytosines by unmethylated ones (15). Interestingly, GADD45 proteins are also known to be involved in stress response (18), which could imply that environmental stress can affect early gonadal development and testosterone production. Increased gonadal sex hormones levels are needed for developmental reprogramming of the hypothalamus in a sexual dimorphic manner, for the development of reproductive organs, and for imprinting of sexual dimorphic behavior. In the prenatal brain of male rodents, it has been shown that aromatase (*Cyp19a1*) readily converts (aromatizes) testosterone into estrogen (E2) that is responsible for imprinting male-typical behavior (19,20). During this period, increase in the transcription-activating mark histone 3 (H3) acetylation is found at the *Cyp19a1* gene in males, coinciding with their testosterone surge (21).

Another critical window for hormonal influence is the neonatal period when sex-differentiated development of the hypothalamus occurs. It has been shown that variations in transient hormonal surges associated with maternal care given with a preference to male over female neonatal pups has lasting effects on DNA methylation of the estrogen receptor alpha (ERα) promoter in the hypothalamus and thus on adult sexual behavior (22,23).

Puberty

The initiation of mammalian puberty is orchestrated by a myriad of complex interactions involving different cell types and organs that activate large and interconnected gene networks. Although the molecular mechanisms are still largely obscure, from a neuronal perspective it is known that puberty is triggered by trans-synaptic (24,25) and glial (26) interactions with hypothalamic neurons that release GnRH. Kisseptins are neuropeptides that have a major role in GnRH release. Kisspeptins are transcribed from the *KISS1* gene and bind to the kisseptin receptor (*GPR54/KISS1R*) on GnRH neurons of the hypothalamus (24,27,28). GnRH, in turn, triggers the release of LH and FSH from the anterior pituitary, leading to downstream effects in hormonal levels related to pubertal progression, development of secondary sexual characteristics, and ovulation in females. De-methylation of a regulatory region of the *GNRH* gene seems to be one of the mechanisms of regulation of GnRH release during puberty (29).

Both *KISS1* and *GNRH* are suggested to be under hormonally dependent epigenetic control. For example, peripubertal increases in gonadal estrogen (E2) levels (in female rodents) promote the binding of the estrogen receptor alpha (ERα) to the *Kiss1* promoter (30,31). This binding, which appears to be mediated by reduced H3 acetylation, promotes a peripubertal GnRH surge (30,31). Interestingly, as mentioned above, *ERα* is itself under epigenetic control, with both DNA methylation (32) and histone deacetylase (HDAC) modifications in the promoter (21) being fundamental in regulating *ERα* expression and sexual development.

Adulthood

Increasing evidence points toward nuclear receptor (NR) transcription factors, including the sex hormone receptors, as having an important role in epigenetic regulation of gene expression. NRs can recruit both chromatin-remodeling co-activators with histone acetylase (HAT) and deacetylase (HDAC) activities (33,34) and direct *de novo* DNA methylation and de-methylation to regulatory regions (34,35). The mechanisms underlying NR-induced DNA de-methylation is still unclear, however, recent reports show evidence that at least ERα (36), ERβ (37), retinoic acid receptor alpha (RARα) (38), and androgen receptor (AR) (39) can direct DNA de-methylation to specific genomic loci by interacting with thymine DNA glycosylase (TDG). TDG belongs to the base excision repair machinery and is part of the final step in DNA de-methylation by replacing deaminated methylcytosines to unmethylated cytosines. In the case of ERα, the TDG-ERα interaction is dependent on E2 activation (36), however, for ERβ this does not seem to be the case (37). Instead, it can be speculated that antagonistic ligands may be more important in modulating the interaction between ERβ and TDG. In view of the essential roles that sex hormones play in sexual differentiation and reproduction, deregulations in sex hormone signaling may directly impose lasting effects on the epigenome, not only in the affected individual, but also in the offspring.

In females, the dynamic changes in sex-hormone levels during the menstrual cycle, for example fluctuating E2 levels, appear to occur through the involvement of hormonal action on epigenetic mechanisms. These dynamic hormonal changes are regulated by the equally dynamic expression of *Cyp19a1* and the steroidogenic acute regulatory protein (*Star*), which is also involved in progesterone synthesis (40). Interestingly, the action of both enzymes, which are constantly unmethylated, are under the control of LH surges that trigger highly dynamic histone marks within their promoter regions (41–43). While *Cyp19a1* is rapidly suppressed after the LH surge, *Star* is rapidly upregulated in relation to luteinization following ovulation.

In adult males, spermatogenesis is dependent on high levels of free testosterone and is sensitive to drops in these levels (44). Additionally, spermatogenesis relies heavily on proper DNA methylation and chromatin remodeling of regulatory elements of testis genes (45,46,47). Interestingly, testosterone and FSH differentially affect sperm chromatin remodeling through epigenetic mechanisms and transcription factors that ultimately hamper the replacement of histones with protamines (48). Testosterone deficits interfere with the expression of proteins involved in the biogenesis of small non-coding RNAs, the levels of histone deacetylases (HDAC1 and 6), and generate modifications in histones such as h2b and the testis specific th3 (48). FSH deficits, in turn, affect the turnover of ubiquitylated histones and inhibit DNA repair mechanisms, leading to sperm DNA damage (48).

6.4 ENVIRONMENTAL EPIGENETICS: THE STUDY OF HOW EXTRINSIC FACTORS INFLUENCE EPIGENETIC MARKS

The terms "Environmental Epigenetics" and "Environmental Epigenomics" were first mentioned in the 2007 review article "Environmental Epigenomics and Disease Susceptibility" by Jirtle and Skinner (49). At the time, this review summarized many of the important studies that led to the conceptual definition of the terms. The trend of correlating environmental exposures and epigenetic changes, however, started much earlier, and it could be consider that the seminal paper was the 1998 review "Epigenetics and Epimutagens: Some New Perspectives on Cancer, Germline Effects and Endocrine Disrupters" by MacPhee (50). In this paper, MacPhee argues that previously published estrogen-dependent effects on the expression and DNA methylation of the vitellogenin promoter in laying hens (51) could be mimicked by the action of endocrine disruptors (EDCs), that is, compounds that alter the function of the endocrine system in organisms. In a visionary fashion, MacPhee stated: "*Other epigenetic changes (inappropriate methylation, generalised hypomethylation) associated with exposure to environmental agents may also be recognised more readily in the future.*" Three years later, John McLachlan also suggested that estrogens or endocrine disrupting chemicals could play a role in the programming or imprinting of genes through persistent changes in DNA methylation (52).

In the following years, endocrine disruptors started to become the main environmental influence known to affect epigenetic changes, and have since been one of the strongest drivers of the field of "Environmental Epigenetics." Meanwhile, other environmental factors started to be studied and gained importance in relation to epigenetic effects. These include pharmacological compounds known as demethylating agents, nutritional compounds that provide the substrate needed (methyl groups) for DNA methylation reactions, or inorganic chemicals.

Nowadays most scientists in related disciplines would agree that environmental factors are able to influence the establishment of epigenetic mechanisms, and that this process can occur through many different biological pathways. Here we describe four groups of environmental compounds for which there is abundant evidence of related epigenetic effects: endocrine disruptors; nutritional factors; pharmacological compounds; inorganic compounds.

Endocrine Disruptors and Epigenetic Changes

We have recently extensively reviewed the literature related to the connection between EDCs and epigenetic changes (53). This connection, as previously mentioned, has been a driving force for the field of environmental epigenetics, especially regarding transgenerational effects. Nowadays, the literature reporting actions of EDCs on epigenetic mechanisms is extensive. For example, EDCs are shown to regulate numerous endocrine related genes through DNA methylation, which includes well-known receptors such as to estrogen, progesterone, glucocorticoids, mineralocorticoids, retinoic acid, oxytocin, follicle-stimulating hormone, thyroid-stimulating hormone, and the insulin-like growth factor (53). EDCs reported to induce epigenetic effects include DES, BPA, Benzo[a]pyrene, Vinclozolin, n-butylparaben, DEHP, PCBs, and TCDD, among others (53).

Although the exact mechanism by which EDC promote epigenetic changes is still not fully elucidated, recent research has given hints on potential mechanisms. Because EDCs mimic the action of endogenous hormones, they can, in theory, interfere with endocrine response both at the physiological and molecular levels. Such interference is reported to have reproductive effects. Well-known examples of detrimental reproductive effects are those produced by exposures to DES (54), BPA (55), and vinclozolin (56). Once EDCs bind to cytosolic receptors that belong to the nuclear hormone receptors (NHRs) superfamily, either they can trigger responses through the classical genomic pathway or through the non-genomic pathway (57). The genomic pathway involves nuclear translocation and the further binding of the ligand-activated hormone receptors to hormone-responsive elements in the genome, while the non-genomic pathway involves the rapid and transient induction of membrane-initiated signaling pathways that activate kinase cascades (57). EDCs appear to act on hormone receptors through both pathways (57). EDCs can also mimic hormonal action that takes place directly on genomic regions known as "response elements" such as the estrogen response element (ERE) (58,59). For example, Bhan et al. (60) have shown that the binding of EDCs to an ERE within the promoter of a non-coding RNA (HOTAIR) enables the binding of histones methylases that will modify the chromatin and activate gene expression (60).

Nutritional Factors and Epigenetic Changes

Nutrition is a critical environmental component influencing the epigenome. This is particularly important for DNA methylation, which requires the presence of methyl-group substrates, commonly derived from the diet. Dietary sources of methyl groups include folic acid, betaine, zinc, and vitamin B_{12}, which ultimately participate in the metabolism of methionine and S-adenosil methionine (SAM) (61). SAM is formed from methyl groups derived from choline, methionine or methyl-tetrahydrofolate, and is the primary methyl donor for the various methyltransferase enzymes in organisms (62). The amount of folates in the diet can directly influence their levels in the blood (63).

Possibly the best known animal model for studying the effects of dietary methyl donors on DNA methylation is the agouti mouse. Using this model, changes in methylation in the Avy allele can be easily detected through changes in the coat color. Specifically, the level of DNA methylation in an intracisternal A particle (IAP) retro-transposon located upstream of the Avy allele correlates with coat color shifts from yellow-agouti to yellow (64). Changes in maternal consumption of methyl groups lead to coat color variations in the offspring, which correlates with the methylation status of the Avy allele (64,65). Other experiments have taken advantage of other properties of the Avy allele, such as its association with obesity (66,67).

Another model exploiting phenotypic traits to reflect DNA methylation in IAP elements uses IAPs located upstream of the promoter of Axin fused. In this case, high Axin fused DNA methylation in the tail is associated with a straight tail phenotype, while low levels correlate with a kinky tail phenotype (68). Both tail axin fused DNA methylation and kinky/straight phenotype correlate with the pre- and post-natal availability of methyl groups.

Nutritional factors also influence the expression of Dnmts. In humans, increased *DNMT1* (the maintenance Dnmt) expression in observed in cervical intraepithelial neoplasia samples after mandatory fortification of grain products with folic acid in the United States (69). Concordantly, Dnmt1 has been shown to be reduced in the liver of rat offspring born to protein-restricted mothers (70). In addition to DNA methylation, dietary compounds have also been implicated in the modulation of other epigenetic systems, such as histone modifications (71) and non-coding RNAs (72).

In addition to folate groups, dietary flavonoids have also been associated with epigenetic changes. Flavonoids (or isoflavones) is a class of plant compounds that elicit estrogenic actions in animals (73), and hence are also called phytoestrogens. Dietary intake of phytoestrogens is known to produce reproductive effects in mammals (74–77) including humans (78), where isoflavones are reported to be transferred from mother to child through breastfeeding (79).

Initial experiments showed that administration of the phytoestrogens coumestrol and equol to newborn mice inactivated the proto-oncogene H-ras through increased DNA methylation (80). Later, it has been shown that consumption of high doses of the phytoestrogen genistein by 8-week-old mice induces altered DNA methylation patterns (81), while neonatal exposure of females to high genistein levels results in tissue-specific hypermethylation in the gene Nsbp1 (nucleosomal binding protein) in the uterus (82). Also in mice, gender-specific changes in DNA methylation of the Acta1 promoter in the liver are observed in response to a diet rich in the phytoestrogens genistein and daidzein (83). The Agouti mouse model has also been used to evidence the epigenetic effects of phytoestrogens. With this model, hypomethylation of the Avy allele induced by maternal exposure to BPA was shown to be inhibited by maternal dietary supplementation with either methyl-donors or genistein (84). Table 6.1 summarizes studies that investigate epigenetic effects induced via nutrition.

The epigenomic effects of dietary phytoestrogens are not limited to DNA methylation. In prostate cancer, genistein has a protective effect that takes place through the activation of tumor suppressor genes by histone modifications and chromatin remodeling (85). In breast cancer cells, genistein, in addition to reducing the expression of Dnmts, inhibits the

TABLE 6.1   Nutritional Factors and Epigenetic Changes

Nutritional Factor	Experimental Model	Effect	References
Methyl supplemented maternal diet	Mouse (agouti)	Increased longevity and DNA methylation in LTR repeats in liver and kidney	[64]
Methyl supplemented maternal diet	Mouse (agouti)	Altered coat color in mice exposed as embryos and their offspring. Coat color is dependent on methylation levels at the Avy allele	[65]
Maternal dietary genistein	Mouse (agouti)	Altered coat color in mice exposed as embryos and DNA methylation in LTR repeats in many tissues	[66]
Methyl supplemented maternal diet	Mouse (axin fu)	Increased DNA methylation in the Axin-fused allele, and reduction in the incidence of kinky tail phenotype	[68]
Folic acid supplementation	Human samples of cervical intraepithelial neoplasia	Increased DNMT1 expression	[69]
Dietary genistein	Mouse (C57BL/6J)	DNA methylation differences in a novel gene in prostate	[81]
Dietary genistein and daidzein	Mouse (C3H)	Suppression of gender-specific differences in body weight and in promoter DNA methylation in Acta1 (liver); advanced sexual maturation in females	[83]
Maternal diet with methyl supplementation and genistein	Mouse (agouti)	Neutralization of BPA-induced hypermethylation in Avy alleles	[84]

hTERT (human telomerase reverse transcriptase) gene by promoting hypomethylation in E2F-1 sites (thereby increased E2F-1 binding) and altering methylation in H3K9 and H3K4 histones in its promoter (86).

Pharmacological Compounds and Epigenetic Changes

The first pharmacological agent used to deliberately alter the epigenome was the demethylating agent 5-AzaC. 5-AzaC was initially tested as a treatment against leukemia in mice (87) and is currently approved by the FDA (since 2004) for the chemotherapeutical treatment of the myelodysplastic syndrome (88). In addition to 5-AzaC, there are currently a number of other epigenetic drugs approved for clinical use by the FDA (89): Decitabine (5-aza-2'-deoxycytidine) is also a hypomethylating agent with similar therapeutic applications as 5-AzaC for the treatment of myelodysplastic syndrome; Tranylcypromine and phenelzine are lysine demethylase inhibitors initially approved as anti-depressants, but currently also tested for cancer treatment; Trichostatin-A, Vorinostat, Panobinostat, and Belinostat are HDAC inhibitors (of the hydroxamic acids group) employed in the treatment

TABLE 6.2   Current Approval Status of Pharmacological Agents

Drug (s)	Epigenetic Mechanism	Uses	Approval Status
5-AzaC	DNA methylation	Treatment of myelodysplastic syndrome	FDA approved
Tranylcypromine and phenelzine	Lysine demethylase inhibitors	Anti-depressants	FDA approved
		Cancer treatment	Being tested
Trichostatin-A, Vorinostat, Panobinostat, and Belinostat	Histone deacetylase inhibitors	Treatment of lymphoma and leukemia	FDA approved
Mocetinostat	Histone deacetylase inhibitor	Treatment of myelodysplastic syndrome	FDA approved
Romidepsin	Histone deacetylase inhibitor	Treatment of cutaneous T-cell lymphoma, after patients have had systemic therapy	FDA approved
Miravirsen and RG-101	miRNAs	Treatment of hepatitis C	Clinical trials
MRX34	miRNAs	Treatment of cancer	Clinical trials

of lymphoma and leukemia; Mocetinostat is an HDAC inhibitor from the benzamides group also employed for the treatment of myelodysplastic syndrome; Romidepsin is an HDAC I and II inhibitor with cyclic tetrapeptide antibiotic and antineoplastic activity approved for the treatment of patients with cutaneous T-cell lymphoma, used after they have been administered with systemic therapy (89). In addition, three epigenetic drugs based on the action of miRNAs have entered clinical trials: Miravirsen and RG-101 for the treatment of hepatitis C, and MRX34 for the treatment of cancer (89). Table 6.2 summarizes the current status of pharmacological agents that alter the epigenome.

Inorganic Compounds and Epigenetic Changes

Special attention is currently given to the epigenetic effects of inorganic compounds due to increasing knowledge about the consequences of exposure of human populations to heavy metals. One of the first inorganic elements that has been related with epigenetic effects is arsenic, due to its reported role in the metabolism of methyl groups (90). In mice in which hepatocellular carcinoma has been induced by exposure to arsenic in utero, altered estrogen signaling plays a role, in which arsenic induces overexpression of ERα and hypomethylation in regions of the ERα promoter in the liver (91). In mouse Leydig (MLTC-1) cells arsenic exposure induces upregulation of 3β-HSD (3β-hydroxysteroid dehydrogenase) through the suppression of histone H3K9 di- and tri-methylation (92). Another inorganic element of recent concern is cadmium due to its carcinogenic properties and adverse health effects in relation to smoking. In humans, high cadmium levels detected in urine samples (associated with smoking status) correlated with hypomethylation in MGMT gene independent of gender, hypomethylation in MT2A and DNMT3B in women, and LINE-1 hypermethylation in men (93). In human bronchial epithelial cells that undergo cadmium-induced malignant transformation, Dnmts get progressively overexpressed, which increases global DNA methylation, while the expression of DNA repair genes is progressively reduced (94).

6.5 CONCLUDING REMARKS

Timely epigenetic events mediate proper development in organisms and contribute to the formation of healthy individuals. These events are highly plastic, allowing the organism to cope with variations in its surrounding environment. However, such plasticity also implies that developmental windows of increased epigenetic remodeling may be sensitive to the action of environmental exposures that will generate detrimental outcomes. Nutritional factors, EDCs (man-made or natural) or various pharmacological agents are currently known to act on epigenetic processes, thereby interfering with the epigenetic machineries. In parallel, it is important to consider the known detrimental effects EDCs exert on reproduction, such as those generated by exposure to BPA and phytoestrogens. Increasing evidence points toward endocrine signaling, particularly signaling involving sex hormones, as being very sensitive to epigenetic remodeling by extrinsic factors. This is of special concern since sex-hormone signaling is not only needed for the normal functioning of the adult organism but also for its reproductive ability. Future research on the interaction between intrinsic and extrinsic epigenetic regulation is therefore warranted.

REFERENCES

1. Jablonka E, Lamb MJ. The changing concept of epigenetics. *Ann N Y Acad Sci.* 2002;981:82–96.
2. Skinner MK, Manikkam M, Guerrero-Bosagna C. Epigenetic transgenerational actions of environmental factors in disease etiology. *Trends Endocrinol Metab.* 2010;21(4):214–22.
3. Reik W, Dean W, Walter J. Epigenetic reprogramming in mammalian development. *Science.* 2001;293(5532):1089–93.
4. Lees-Murdock DJ, Walsh CP. DNA methylation reprogramming in the germ line. *Epigenetics.* 2008;3(1):5–13.
5. Hackett JA, Surani MA. Beyond DNA: Programming and inheritance of parental methylomes. *Cell.* 2013;153(4):737–9.
6. Denisenko O, Lucas ES, Sun C et al. Regulation of ribosomal RNA expression across the lifespan is fine-tuned by maternal diet before implantation. *Biochim Biophys Acta.* 2016;1859(7):906–13.
7. Wu Q, Ohsako S, Ishimura R et al. Exposure of mouse preimplantation embryos to 2,3,7,8-tetrachlorodibenzo-p-dioxin (TCDD) alters the methylation status of imprinted genes H19 and Igf2. *Biol Reprod.* 2004;70(6):1790–7.
8. Guerrero-Bosagna C, Covert TR, Haque MM et al. Epigenetic transgenerational inheritance of vinclozolin induced mouse adult onset disease and associated sperm epigenome biomarkers. *Reprod Toxicol.* 2012;34(4):694–707.
9. Guerrero-Bosagna C, Settles M, Lucker B, Skinner MK. Epigenetic transgenerational actions of vinclozolin on promoter regions of the sperm epigenome. *PLoS One.* 2010;5(9).

10. Manikkam M, Guerrero-Bosagna C, Tracey R et al. Transgenerational actions of environmental compounds on reproductive disease and identification of epigenetic biomarkers of ancestral exposures. *PLoS One.* 2012;7(2):e31901.

11. Tang WW, Kobayashi T, Irie N et al. Specification and epigenetic programming of the human germ line. *Nat Rev Genet.* 2016;17(10):585–600.

12. Spiller C, Koopman P, Bowles J. Sex determination in the mammalian germline. *Annu Rev Genet.* 2017;51:265–285.

13. Yosefzon Y, David C, Tsukerman A et al. An epigenetic switch repressing Tet1 in gonadotropes activates the reproductive axis. *Proc Natl Acad Sci USA.* 2017;114(38):10131–6.

14. Dawlaty MM, Breiling A, Le T et al. Combined deficiency of Tet1 and Tet2 causes epigenetic abnormalities but is compatible with postnatal development. *Developmental Cell.* 2013;24(3):310–23.

15. Tachibana M. Epigenetic regulation of mammalian sex determination. *J Med Invest.* 2015;62(1–2):19–23.

16. Varshney M, Nalvarte I. Genes, gender, environment, and novel functions of estrogen receptor beta in the susceptibility to neurodevelopmental disorders. *Brain Sciences.* 2017;7(3).

17. Nishino K, Hattori N, Tanaka S, Shiota K. DNA methylation-mediated control of Sry gene expression in mouse gonadal development. *J Biol Chem.* 2004;279(21):22306–13.

18. Liebermann DA, Tront JS, Sha X et al. Gadd45 stress sensors in malignancy and leukemia. *Crit Rev Oncog.* 2011;16(1–2):129–40.

19. Juntti SA, Tollkuhn J, Wu MV et al. The androgen receptor governs the execution, but not programming, of male sexual and territorial behaviors. *Neuron.* 2010;66(2):260–72.

20. Wu MV, Manoli DS, Fraser EJ et al. Estrogen masculinizes neural pathways and sex-specific behaviors. *Cell.* 2009;139(1):61–72.

21. Matsuda KI, Mori H, Nugent BM et al. Histone deacetylation during brain development is essential for permanent masculinization of sexual behavior. *Endocrinology.* 2011;152(7):2760–7.

22. Lauber AH, Mobbs CV, Muramatsu M, Pfaff DW. Estrogen receptor messenger RNA expression in rat hypothalamus as a function of genetic sex and estrogen dose. *Endocrinology.* 1991;129(6):3180–6.

23. McCarthy MM, Auger AP, Bale TL et al. The epigenetics of sex differences in the brain. *J Neurosci.* 2009;29(41):12815–23.

24. Oakley AE, Clifton DK, Steiner RA. Kisspeptin signaling in the brain. *Endocr Rev.* 2009;30(6):713–43.

25. Terasawa E, Fernandez DL. Neurobiological mechanisms of the onset of puberty in primates. *Endocr Rev.* 2001;22(1):111–51.

26. Prevot V. Glial-neuronal-endothelial interactions are involved in the control of GnRH secretion. *J Neuroendocrinol.* 2002;14(3):247–55.

27. de Roux N, Genin E, Carel JC et al. Hypogonadotropic hypogonadism due to loss of function of the KISS1-derived peptide receptor GPR54. *Proc Natl Acad Sci USA.* 2003;100(19):10972–6.

28. Seminara SB, Messager S, Chatzidaki EE et al. The GPR54 gene as a regulator of puberty. *N Engl J Med.* 2003;349(17):1614–27.

29. Kurian JR, Keen KL, Terasawa E. Epigenetic changes coincide with *in vitro* primate GnRH neuronal maturation. *Endocrinology.* 2010;151(11):5359–68.

30. Lomniczi A, Loche A, Castellano JM et al. Epigenetic control of female puberty. *Nat Neurosci.* 2013;16(3):281–9.

31. Tomikawa J, Uenoyama Y, Ozawa M et al. Epigenetic regulation of Kiss1 gene expression mediating estrogen-positive feedback action in the mouse brain. *Proc Natl Acad Sci USA.* 2012;109(20):E1294–301.

32. Kurian JR, Olesen KM, Auger AP. Sex differences in epigenetic regulation of the estrogen receptor-alpha promoter within the developing preoptic area. *Endocrinology.* 2010;151(5):2297–305.

33. Martens JHA, Rao NAS, Stunnenberg HG. Genome-wide interplay of nuclear receptors with the epigenome. *Biochimica et Biophysica Acta (BBA) - Molecular Basis of Disease.* 2011;1812(8):818–23.

34. Romagnolo DF, Zempleni J, Selmin OI. Nuclear receptors and epigenetic regulation: Opportunities for nutritional targeting and disease prevention. *Advances in Nutrition.* 2014;5(4):373–85.

35. Metivier R, Gallais R, Tiffoche C et al. Cyclical DNA methylation of a transcriptionally active promoter. *Nature.* 2008;452(7183):45–50.

36. Chen D, Lucey MJ, Phoenix F et al. T:G mismatch-specific thymine-DNA glycosylase potentiates transcription of estrogen-regulated genes through direct interaction with estrogen receptor alpha. *J Biol Chem.* 2003;278(40):38586–92.

37. Liu Y, Duong W, Krawczyk C et al. Oestrogen receptor beta regulates epigenetic patterns at specific genomic loci through interaction with thymine DNA glycosylase. *Epigenetics & Chromatin.* 2016;9:7.

38. Leger H, Smet-Nocca C, Attmane-Elakeb A et al. A TDG/CBP/RARalpha ternary complex mediates the retinoic acid-dependent expression of DNA methylation-sensitive genes. *Genomics Proteomics Bioinformatics.* 2014;12(1):8–18.

39. Dhiman VK, Attwood K, Campbell MJ, Smiraglia DJ. Hormone stimulation of androgen receptor mediates dynamic changes in DNA methylation patterns at regulatory elements. *Oncotarget.* 2015;6(40):42575–89.

40. Sugino N. Molecular mechanisms of luteinization. *Obstet Gynecol Sci.* 2014;57(2):93–101.

41. Christenson LK, Stouffer RL, Strauss JF 3rd. Quantitative analysis of the hormone-induced hyperacetylation of histone H3 associated with the steroidogenic acute regulatory protein gene promoter. *J Biol Chem.* 2001;276(29):27392–9.

42. Hiroi H, Christenson LK, Chang L et al. Temporal and spatial changes in transcription factor binding and histone modifications at the steroidogenic acute regulatory protein (stAR) locus associated with stAR transcription. *Mol Endocrinol.* 2004;18(4):791–806.

43. Stocco C. Aromatase expression in the ovary: Hormonal and molecular regulation. *Steroids.* 2008;73(5):473–87.

44. Zirkin BR, Santulli R, Awoniyi CA, Ewing LL. Maintenance of advanced spermatogenic cells in the adult rat testis: Quantitative relationship to testosterone concentration within the testis. *Endocrinology.* 1989;124(6):3043–9.

45. Stuppia L, Franzago M, Ballerini P et al. Epigenetics and male reproduction: The consequences of paternal lifestyle on fertility, embryo development, and children lifetime health. *Clin Epigenetics.* 2015;7:120.

46. Rajender S, Avery K, Agarwal A. Epigenetics, spermatogenesis, and male infertility. *Mutat Res.* 2011;727(3):62–71.

47. Vlachogiannis G, Niederhuth CE, Tuna S et al. *The Dnmt3L ADD Domain Controls Cytosine Methylation Establishment during Spermatogenesis.* Cell reports. 2015.

48. Gill-Sharma MK, Choudhuri J, Ansari MA, D'Souza S. Putative molecular mechanism underlying sperm chromatin remodelling is regulated by reproductive hormones. *Clin Epigenetics.* 2012;4(1):23.

49. Jirtle RL, Skinner MK. Environmental epigenomics and disease susceptibility. *Nat Rev Genet.* 2007;8(4):253–62.

50. MacPhee DG. Epigenetics and epimutagens: Some new perspectives on cancer, germ line effects and endocrine disrupters. *Mutat Res.* 1998;400(1–2):369–79.

51. Wilks A, Seldran M, Jost JP. An estrogen-dependent demethylation at the 5' end of the chicken vitellogenin gene is independent of DNA synthesis. *Nucleic Acids Res.* 1984;12(2):1163–77.

52. McLachlan JA. Environmental signaling: What embryos and evolution teach us about endocrine disrupting chemicals. *Endocr Rev.* 2001;22(3):319–41.

53. Jacobs M, Marczylo E, Guerrero-Bosagna C, Rüegg J. Marked for life: Epigenetic effects of endocrine disrupting chemicals. *Annu Rev Environ Resour.* 2017;42:105–60.

54. Newbold RR, Hanson RB, Jefferson WN et al. Proliferative lesions and reproductive tract tumors in male descendants of mice exposed developmentally to diethylstilbestrol. *Carcinogenesis.* 2000;21(7):1355–63.

55. Salian S, Doshi T, Vanage G. Perinatal exposure of rats to Bisphenol A affects fertility of male offspring-an overview. *Reproductive toxicology.* 2011;31(3):359–62.

56. Uzumcu M, Suzuki H, Skinner MK. Effect of the anti-androgenic endocrine disruptor vinclozolin on embryonic testis cord formation and postnatal testis development and function. *Reproductive Toxicology.* 2004;18(6):765–74.

57. Wong RL, Walker CL. Molecular pathways: Environmental estrogens activate nongenomic signaling to developmentally reprogram the epigenome. *Clin Cancer Res.* 2013;19(14):3732–7.

58. Hyder SM, Stancel GM, Nawaz Z et al. Identification of an estrogen response element in the 3'-flanking region of the murine c-fos protooncogene. *J Biol Chem.* 1992;267(25):18047–54.

59. Weisz A, Rosales R. Identification of an estrogen response element upstream of the human c-fos gene that binds the estrogen receptor and the AP-1 transcription factor. *Nucleic Acids Res.* 1990;18(17):5097–106.

60. Bhan A, Mandal SS. Estradiol-induced transcriptional regulation of long non-coding RNA, HOTAIR. *Methods Mol Biol.* 2016;1366:395–412.

61. Van den Veyver IB. Genetic effects of methylation diets. *Annu Rev Nutr.* 2002;22:255–82.

62. Zeisel SH. Epigenetic mechanisms for nutrition determinants of later health outcomes. *Am J Clin Nutr.* 2009;89(5):1488S–93S.

63. Hirsch S, Ronco AM, Guerrero-Bosagna C et al. Methylation status in healthy subjects with normal and high serum folate concentration. *Nutrition.* 2008;24(11–12):1103–9.

64. Cooney CA, Dave AA, Wolff GL. Maternal methyl supplements in mice affect epigenetic variation and DNA methylation of offspring. *J Nutr.* 2002;132(8 Suppl):2393S–400S.

65. Cropley JE, Suter CM, Beckman KB, Martin DI. Germ-line epigenetic modification of the murine Avy allele by nutritional supplementation. *Proc Natl Acad Sci USA.* 2006;103(46):17308–12.

66. Dolinoy DC, Weidman JR, Waterland RA, Jirtle RL. Maternal genistein alters coat color and protects Avy mouse offspring from obesity by modifying the fetal epigenome. *Environ Health Perspect.* 2006;114(4):567–72.

67. Yen TT, Gill AM, Frigeri LG et al. Obesity, diabetes, and neoplasia in yellow A(vy)/- mice: Ectopic expression of the agouti gene. *Faseb J.* 1994;8(8):479–88.

68. Waterland RA, Dolinoy DC, Lin JR et al. Maternal methyl supplements increase offspring DNA methylation at Axin Fused. *Genesis.* 2006;44(9):401–6.

69. Piyathilake CJ, Celedonio JE, Macaluso M et al. Mandatory fortification with folic acid in the United States is associated with increased expression of DNA methyltransferase-1 in the cervix. *Nutrition.* 2008;24(1):94–9.

70. Lillycrop KA, Slater-Jefferies JL, Hanson MA et al. Induction of altered epigenetic regulation of the hepatic glucocorticoid receptor in the offspring of rats fed a protein-restricted diet during pregnancy suggests that reduced DNA methyltransferase-1 expression is involved in impaired DNA methylation and changes in histone modifications. *Br J Nutr.* 2007;97(6):1064–73.

71. Delage B, Dashwood RH. Dietary manipulation of histone structure and function. *Annu Rev Nutr.* 2008;28:347–66.

72. Quintanilha BJ, Reis BZ, Duarte GBS et al. Nutrimiromics: Role of microRNAs and nutrition in modulating inflammation and chronic diseases. *Nutrients.* 2017;9(11).

73. Liggins J, Bluck LJ, Runswick S et al. Daidzein and genistein contents of vegetables. *Br J Nutr.* 2000;84(5):717–25.

74. Adams NR. A changed responsiveness to oestrogen in ewes with clover disease. *J Reprod Fertil Suppl.* 1981;30:223–30.

75. Adams NR, Hearnshaw H, Oldham CM. Abnormal function of the corpus luteum in some ewes with phyto-oestrogenic infertility. *Aust J Biol Sci.* 1981;34(1):61–5.

76. Gallo D, Cantelmo F, Distefano M et al. Reproductive effects of dietary soy in female Wistar rats. *Food Chem Toxicol.* 1999;37(5):493–502.

77. Santell RC, Chang YC, Nair MG, Helferich WG. Dietary genistein exerts estrogenic effects upon the uterus, mammary gland and the hypothalamic/pituitary axis in rats. *J Nutr.* 1997;127(2):263–9.

78. Pino AM, Valladares LE, Palma MA et al. Dietary isoflavones affect sex hormone-binding globulin levels in postmenopausal women. *J Clin Endocrinol Metab.* 2000;85(8):2797–800.

79. Franke AA, Halm BM, Custer LJ et al. Isoflavones in breastfed infants after mothers consume soy. *Am J Clin Nutr.* 2006;84(2):406–13.

80. Lyn-Cook BD, Blann E, Payne PW et al. Methylation profile and amplification of proto-oncogenes in rat pancreas induced with phytoestrogens. *Proc Soc Exp Biol Med.* 1995;208(1):116–9.

81. Day JK, Bauer AM, DesBordes C et al. Genistein alters methylation patterns in mice. *J Nutr.* 2002;132(8 Suppl):2419S–23S.

82. Tang WY, Newbold R, Mardilovich K et al. Persistent hypomethylation in the promoter of nucleosomal binding protein 1 (Nsbp1) correlates with overexpression of Nsbp1 in mouse uteri neonatally exposed to diethylstilbestrol or genistein. *Endocrinology.* 2008;149(12):5922–31.

83. Guerrero-Bosagna CM, Sabat P, Valdovinos FS et al. Epigenetic and phenotypic changes result from a continuous pre and post natal dietary exposure to phytoestrogens in an experimental population of mice. *BMC Physiol.* 2008;8:17.

84. Dolinoy DC, Huang D, Jirtle RL. Maternal nutrient supplementation counteracts bisphenol A-induced DNA hypomethylation in early development. *Proc Natl Acad Sci USA.* 2007;104:13056–61.

85. Majid S, Kikuno N, Nelles J et al. Genistein induces the p21WAF1/CIP1 and p16INK4a tumor suppressor genes in prostate cancer cells by epigenetic mechanisms involving active chromatin modification. *Cancer Res.* 2008;68(8):2736–44.

86. Li Y, Liu L, Andrews LG, Tollefsbol TO. Genistein depletes telomerase activity through cross-talk between genetic and epigenetic mechanisms. *Int J Cancer.* 2009;125(2):286–96.

87. Neil GL, Moxley TE, Kuentzel SL et al. Enhancement by tetrahydrouridine (NSC-112907) of the oral activity of 5-azacytidine (NSC-102816) in L1210 leukemic mice. *Cancer Chemother Rep.* 1975;59(3):459–65.

88. Kaminskas E, Farrell AT, Wang YC et al. FDA drug approval summary: Azacitidine (5-azacytidine, Vidaza) for injectable suspension. *Oncologist.* 2005;10(3):176–82.

89. Hodjat M, Rahmani S, Khan F et al. Environmental toxicants, incidence of degenerative diseases, and therapies from the epigenetic point of view. *Arch Toxicol.* 2017;91(7):2577–97.

90. Vahter ME. Interactions between arsenic-induced toxicity and nutrition in early life. *J Nutr.* 2007;137(12):2798–804.

91. Waalkes MP, Liu J, Chen H et al. Estrogen signaling in livers of male mice with hepatocellular carcinoma induced by exposure to arsenic in utero. *J Natl Cancer Inst.* 2004;96(6):466–74.

92. Alamdar A, Xi G, Huang Q et al. Arsenic activates the expression of 3beta-HSD in mouse Leydig cells through repression of histone H3K9 methylation. *Toxicol Appl Pharmacol.* 2017;326:7–14.

93. Virani S, Rentschler KM, Nishijo M et al. DNA methylation is differentially associated with environmental cadmium exposure based on sex and smoking status. *Chemosphere.* 2016;145:284–90.

94. Zhou ZH, Lei YX, Wang CX. Analysis of aberrant methylation in DNA repair genes during malignant transformation of human bronchial epithelial cells induced by cadmium. *Toxicol Sci.* 2012;125(2):412–7.

CHAPTER 7

Epigenetic and Assisted Reproduction Epidemiological Studies

Thomas Eggermann

CONTENTS

7.1 INTRODUCTION

Assisted reproductive technologies (ART), defined as treatments handling at least one gamete outside the body, include procedures such as *in vitro* fertilization (IVF) and intracytoplasmic sperm injection (ICSI). In industrialized countries, ART accounts for 1%–3% of all births in industrialized countries. In general, ART techniques are regarded as safe, but a number of reports of patients with imprinting disorders (ImpDis) born after ART has raised the question for a causal relationship.

The term "Imprinting disorders" (ImpDis) refers to a molecularly defined group of congenital diseases which are characterized by similar types of molecular alterations of imprinted genes (Figure 7.1). These mutations and epimutations disturb the fine-tuned balance of the affected imprinted genes. However, with some exceptions the resulting pathomechanisms and functional links to the resulting clinical pictures are often unknown.

7.2 MOLECULAR CHANGES IN IMPRINTING DISORDERS

In the majority of ImpDis, specific imprinted loci are affected by (epi)mutations (Table 7.1), but in some disorders more than one differentially methylated regions (DMRs) can be affected. This locus heterogeneity can comprise two adjacent loci (e.g., ICR1 and ICR2 in 11p15 in the case of Beckwith-Wiedemann syndrome) or two loci on different chromosomes (e.g., chromosomes 7 and 11p15 in Silver-Russell syndrome). Furthermore, there are a growing number of reports on patients with molecular disturbances at different DMRs (Multilocus Imprinting Disturbance, MLID, see below).

Though ImpDis are caused by molecular alterations affecting the imprinted gene itself or its expression, they show several deviations from classical Mendelian inheritance.

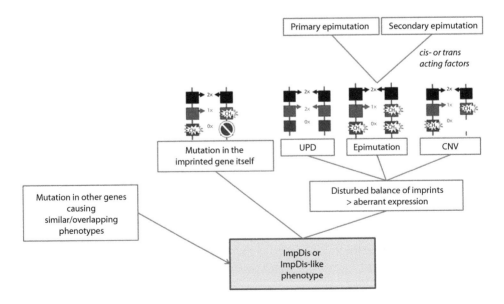

FIGURE 7.1   Types of mutations and epimutations in patients with ImpDis phenotypes.

TABLE 7.1 Overview on the Types and Frequencies of Mutations and Epimutations in ImpDis, Major Clinical Findings, and Numbers of Children Born after ART

Disorder	Chrom.	Molecular Alterations	Frequencies	MLID	Number of Patients Born after ART	Clinical Features
Transient neonatal diabetes mellitus (TNDM) OMIM 601410	6q24	upd(6)pat	41%	–	1	IUGR, transient diabetes, hyperglycemia without ketoacidosis, macroglossia, omphalocele
		dup(6q)	29%	–		
		PLAGL1:alt-TSS-DMR: LOM	30%	50%		
Silver-Russell syndrome (SRS) OMIM 180860	7	upd(7)mat	7%–10%	–		IUGR, PNGR, relative macrocephaly, asymmetry, prominent forehead/triangular face, feeding difficulties
		GRB10 hypermethylation	Single case	–		
		MEST hypermethylation	Single case	–	1	
		CNVs (dup[7p], del[7q])	Single cases	–		
	11p15.5	upd(11)mat	n = 1	–		
		dup(11p15)mat	1%–2%	–		
		H19/IGF2:IG-DMR: LOM	>38%	10%–33%	13	
		CDKN1C mutations	n = 1	–		
		IGF2 mutations	n = 1	–		
Birk-Barel mental retardation OMIM: 612292	8q24.3	KCNK9 mutations	Unknown	–		Intellectual disability, hyperactivity, feeding difficulties, hypotonia, elongated face
Beckwith-Wiedemann syndrome (BWS) OMIM 130650		upd(11)pat	20%	–	1 case?	Pre- and postnatal overgrowth, organomegaly, macroglossia, omphalocele, neonatal hypoglycemia, hemihypertrophy, increased tumour risk
		uniparental diploidy	~10%?	–		
		paternal UPD	~90%	–		
		dup(11p15)pat	1%–2%	–	–	
		H19/IGF2:IG-DMR: GOM	4%	–	–	
		KCNQ1OT1:TSS-DMR: LOM	50%	25%	86	
		CDKN1C mutations	5%	–	–	

(Continued)

TABLE 7.1 (*Continued*) Overview on the Types and Frequencies of Mutations and Epimutations in ImpDis, Major Clinical Findings, and Numbers of Children Born after ART

Disorder	Chrom.	Molecular Alterations	Frequencies	MLID	Number of Patients Born after ART	Clinical Features
Temple syndrome (UPD(14)mat) OMIM 616222	14q32	upd(14)mat	78.4%	–		IUGR,PNGR, hypotonia, Feeding difficulties in infancy, truncal obesity, scoliosis, precocious puberty
		del(14q32)pat	9.8%	–		
		MEG3/DLK1:IG-DMR and *MEG3*:TSS-DMR: LOM	11.7%	–		
Kagami-Ogata syndrome (UPD(14)pat) OMIM 608149		upd(14)pat	65.4%	–		IUGR, polyhydramnion, abdominal, and thoracal wall defects, bell-shaped thorax, coat-hanger ribs
		del(14q32)mat	19.2%	–		
		MEG3/DLK1:IG-DMR and *MEG3*:TSS-DMR: GOM	15.4%			
Angelman syndrome (AS) OMIM 105830	15q11q13	UPD(15)pat	1%–2%	–		Mental retardation, microcephaly, no speech, unmotivated laughing, ataxia, seizures
		del(15q11q13)mat	75%	–	10	
		SNURF:TSS-DMR: LOM	~3%	–	7	
		UBE3A mutations	5%–10%	–		
Prader-Willi syndrome (PWS) OMIM 176270		upd(15)mat	25%–30%	–		PNGR, mental retardation, neonatal hypotonia, hypogenitalism, hypopigmentation, obesity/hyperphagia
		del(15q 11q13)pat	70%–75%	–	Yes	
		SNURF:TSS-DMR: GOM	~1%	1 case		
Precocious puberty OMIM 615346	15q	*MKRN3* mutations	Unknown	–		Precocious puberty (girls: 5.75 years, boys: 8.10 years)
Sporadic Pseudohyper-parathyreoidism Ib OMIM 603233	20q13	upd(20)pat	10%–25%	–		Resistance to PTH and other hormones, Albright hereditary osteodystrophy, subcutaneous ossifications, feeding behavior anomalies, normal growth
		del(20q13)	rare	–		
		GNAS-NESP:TSS-DMR: LOM GNAS-XL:Ex1-DMR: LOM GNAS A/B:TSS-DMR	>60%	12.5%		
Mulchandani-Bhoj-Conlin syndrome (upd(20)mat) OMIM 617352	20	upd(20)mat	Unknown	–		IUGR, PNGR, failure to thrive

Abbreviations: upd(6)pat = paternal uniparental disomy of chromosome 6; LOM = loss of methylation; GOM = gain of methylation; CNVs = copy number variations; IUGR = intrauterine growth retardation; PNGR = postnatal growth retardation.

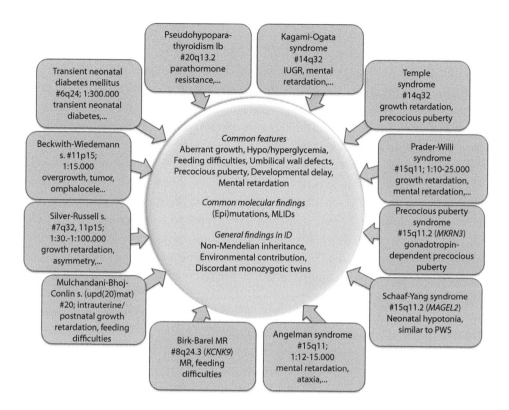

FIGURE 7.2   Common observations in ImpDis. Estimated frequencies in the population are only given for those ImpDis for which data have been suggested.

When familial, inheritance of deletions/duplications and point mutations affecting an imprinted gene is usually autosomal dominant, but the penetrance of the mutation depends on the sex of the parent contributing the affected allele. Typical examples are *CDKN1C* mutations which result in a pathological phenotype only if the active maternal is affected. Genetic counselling becomes even more challenging in case of a chromosomal translocation affecting an imprinted region, which predisposes to a deletion or duplication: In these situations different ImpDis can be expected (1). Another interesting observation in ImpDis is discordant monozygotic twinning (MZ)(2). This discordance is remarkable because MZ twins derive from the same zygote and are therefore genetically identical. It can be explained by epigenetic mosaicism where an early embryo with marked mosaicism between different cells may develop into a single mosaic individual, or if the embryo fragments, it may develop into monozygotic twins with different degrees of epimutation.

7.3 CLINICAL PICTURES

Until now, 12 ImpDis have been identified (Table 7.1, Figure 7.2) based on more or less distinct clinical features or a specific combination of signs. The spectrum of clinical features in ImpDis mainly comprises the following major phenotypic alterations: Aberrant pre- and/or postnatal growth, hypo- or hyperglycemia, abnormal feeding behavior in early childhood and later, umbilical wall defects, developmental delay/behavioral difficulties/ mental retardation, and precocious puberty.

The first identified ImpDis (i.e., Prader-Willi syndrome [PWS]; Angelman syndrome [AS], Beckwith-Wiedemann syndrome [BWS]) have been associated with distinct phenotypes, but in the last years it became obvious that the spectrum of clinical features can be very broad and range from very mild phenotypes to patients with the full clinical picture. Furthermore, the recently identified IDs do not show this distinct separation but clinically overlap with other ImpDis. An example is Temple syndrome (TS14), which has to be considered as a differential diagnosis for Silver-Russell syndrome (SRS) in early childhood and for PWS in late infancy. As a result the distinction between the different ImpDis can be difficult in some situations due to common phenotypic signs and overlapping molecular alterations, and thereby cause problems for accurate diagnosis and targeted treatment. To circumvent this problem clinical scoring systems have been developed for some ImpDis (3), but they fail to detect those patients with only minor or atypical clinical signs, or might indicate another ImpDis than the one which is finally molecularly diagnosed. On molecular level, the clinical heterogeneity can be explained by the mosaic distribution of some (epi) mutations with different ratios of aberrant cells in different tissues (4). Another reason for the clinical overlap between ImpDis is the occurrence of MLID, that is, the altered methylation at different imprinted loci in the same individual (5).

7.4 TYPES OF MUTATIONS AND EPIMUTATIONS IN ImpDis

Four different types of molecular changes associated with ImpDis are currently known (Figure 7.1). Three of them represent genomic alterations, and include large deletions or duplications (copy number variations, CNVs) affecting DMRs, point mutations in the genes themselves, or uniparental disomies (UPDs; i.e., the inheritance of the two homologues from a chromosome pair from the same parent). These alterations of the DNA itself can occur sporadically, or can be inherited, in the latter case a parent-of-origin specific manifestation of the phenotype has to be considered. In contrast, epimutations as the fourth class of molecular alterations in ImpDis are defined as changes which affect the expression of imprinted genes, but not the genomic sequence of the DMR itself. These epimutations either consist of a hypomethylation (loss of methylation, LOM) or a hypermethylation (gain of methylation, GOM), and thereby influence the expression of the imprinted genes. The transitions between point mutations/CNVs and epimutations are fluid, as meanwhile several epimutations have been reported which are the result of a genomic mutation in another chromosomal region or gene influencing the methylation pattern of a DMR. The underlying mutations of these so-called secondary epimutations can either be localized physically close to the altered DMR in *cis* (6), or in a region on another chromosome (e.g., mutations in *ZFP57* genes (7). Molecularly, secondary epimutations cannot be discriminated from primary epimutations as the aberrantly methylated DMR does not show obvious genomic changes. Thus, the identification of an epimutation in an ImpDis patient requires a careful molecular and anamnestic follow-up (e.g., for chromosome 11p15 associated ImpDis [8]), and it becomes increasingly apparent that isolated and sporadic epimutations rather belong to the group of primary epimutations, whereas a familial accumulation and an increased number of spontaneous abortions in a family indicates a genomic cause of the epimutation.

Nearly all ImpDis patients are diagnosed in (early) childhood. However, as already described, the clinical diagnosis is often hampered by the breadth of the phenotypic features which are sometimes subtle, overlapping, and transient. The latter can obscure diagnosis in puberty and adulthood. As a consequence, an unknown number of ImpDis patients are probably either mis- or undiagnosed.

7.5 MULTILOCUS IMPRINTING DEFECTS (MLID)

In a subgroup of patients with primary epimutations, altered imprinting is not restricted to one locus, but affects several DMRs. This MLID has meanwhile been reported in 5 of the 12 ImpDis (Table 7.1). The majority of patients exhibit a specific ImpDis phenotype, e.g., BWS or SRS, and carry the disease-specific epimutations (e.g., ICR2 LOM in BWS or ICR1 LOM in SRS), but additionally other imprinted loci are affected by aberrant methylation. The latter pattern is not disease-specific, and patients with opposite clinical pictures can show similar MLID pattern with the exception of the disease-specific locus. In fact, the reports on MLID are difficult to compare, as the applied methods, the targeted loci and the investigated tissues are not standardized. In fact, the application of genomewide assays and the analysis of a broader spectrum of tissues might circumvent this problem in the future (5,9). However, it is obvious that MLID mainly occurs in BWS and SRS and is detectable in the respective major molecular subgroups (in nearly 25% of ICR2 LOM) and in SRS (up to 10% of ICR1 LOM carriers) (Table 7.1).

The molecular basis for MLID is currently unknown. The observation that different DMRs are affected in MLID but without an obvious pattern of loci indicates that the steps of the imprinting cycle of life (establishment, maintenance or erasure of imprinting markers) are disturbed, but the resulting aberrant methylation show a random distribution. Two causes for MLID are currently discussed. There are an increasing number of reports indicating that genomic mutations play a major in the etiology of MLID. In TNDM and in some SRS and BWS families, genomic mutations in *ZFP57* or *NLRP* genes (*NLRP2, 5, 7*)

TABLE 7.2   Summary of the Studies Focusing on the Link between BWS and ART

References	Country	Number of BWS Patients	Number of BWS Patients Born after Subfertility Treatment	Treatment of Subfertility/ Infertility	Ratio of Children Born after ART among BWS Cohorts	Ratio of Children Born after ART in the General Population°
(31)	USA	65	3	IVF/ICSI	4.6%	0.80%
(32)	United Kingdom	149	6	3 × ICSI, 3 × IvF	4.0%	0.99%
(33)	France	149	6	2 × ICSI, 4 × IVF	4.0%	1.30%
(34)	Australia	37	4	1 × ICSI, 3 × IVF	10.8%	1.13%
(29)	United Kingdom	79	11	5 × ICSI, 1 × IVF, 5 × IT	13.9%	0.80%
(27)	The Netherlands	71	12	6 SP, 4 × IVF/ ICSI, 2 × IT	16.9%	0.92%
(28)	Japan	70	6	1 × ICSI, 5 × IT	8.6%	0.64%–0.98%
(41)	USA	341	19	5 × ICSI, 5 × IVF	5.6%	NR
(37)	UK	11	2	2 × ?	18.2%	NR
(42)	Spain	156	17	15 × IVF, 2 × IT	10.9%	NR
Total		1128	86		7.6%	

Abbreviations: IVF = *In vitro* fertilization; ICSI = intracytoplasmic sperm injection; SP = spontaneously received after time to pregnancy >12 months; IT = infertility treatment without IVF/ICSI (e.g., insemination, ovulation stimulation); NR = not reported.

have meanwhile been identified to be associated with MLID (7,10–12). Additionally, in recent studies on BWS and SRS patients born after assisted reproduction, the frequency of MLID among the 11p15 epimutation carriers has been determined. In fact, a higher number of MLID carriers could be identified in the ART conceived patients than in the general ImpDis cohorts (e.g., 21.2% in BWS patients conceived by ART vs. 4.5% in the general ICR2 LOM cohort (13). However, the number of patients is low and the ascertainment is biased and not standardized. Nevertheless, studies from other mammals indicate an increased incidence of misregulation of multiple imprinted genes in ART cohorts when compared with controls (14). Thus, it can be hypothesized that some steps of the ART procedure predispose to the disturbance of the fine-tuned methylation marking of DMRs. However, the frequency of ART conceived children in the BWS cohorts (Table 7.2) indicates that the 11p15 imprinted loci are particularly prone to these external influences.

7.6 ART AND ImpDis

Since several years it is known that ART technologies can affect the methylation status of some genes in mammals (14,15), and it has been suggested that the establishment and maintenance of DNA methylation of imprinted regions might be disturbed by the

TABLE 7.3   Overview on Reports about SRS Patients with ART

References, Patient	Mode of ART	Phenotype	SRS-Specific Epimutation	MLID[a]
(19) Patient 1	IVF/ICSI	Classical SRS	ND	ND
(19) Patient 2	IVF/ICSI	Classical SRS	ND	ND
(43)	IVF/ICSI	SRS-like	ICR1 LOM	ND
(40)	IVF	Classical SRS +	MEST GOM	ND
(44)	IVF	Classical SRS +	ND	ND
(45)	IVF	Classical SRS	ICR1 LOM	ND
(46)	IVF/ICSI	Classical SRS	ICR1 LOM	ND
(28) Patient 1	IVF	Classical SRS	ICR1 LOM	GOM/LOM at different DMRs
(28) Patient 2	IVF	Classical SRS	ICR1 LOM	No
(28) Patient 3	IVF	Classical SRS	ICR1 LOM	GOM at PLAGL1 DMR
(28) Patient 4	IVF	Classical SRS	ICR1 LOM	GOM at GRB10 DMR
(28) Patient 5	IVF	Classical SRS	ICR1 LOM	GOM at INPP5F DMR
(47)	ICSI	Classical SRS	ICR1 LOM	No
(37)	ART	SRS	ICR1 LOM	No
(37)	ART	SRS	ICR1 LOM	No
(37)	ART	SRS	ICR1 LOM	No

Abbreviations: IVF = *In vitro* fertilization; ICSI = intracytoplasmic sperm injection; ND = not determined.
[a] The different studies used different methods and tissues, therefore the MLID results are hardly comparable.

use of fertility drugs as well as by *in vitro* culture of embryos. On the other hand, it has been postulated that the infertility itself might be regarded as a risk factor for congenital anomalies, including ImpDis (16).

The first indication for a link between ART and human imprinting disorders were the reports of two children born after ICSI with Angelman syndrome (AS) and an imprinting defect, which represents a rare molecular change in AS (17,18) (Table 7.1). At the same time, the first reports on epimutations in 11p15 in patients with BWS (Table 7.2) and SRS were published (19) (Table 7.3), indicating an increased frequency of ART conceived children in these cohorts. However, the comparison of these studies is hampered because their methodologies differed in the inclusion criteria for ImpDis. Some studies included patients with clinical diagnoses, but without the application of a standardized clinical questionnaire, other groups considered cases with a molecularly confirmed ImpDis only. Furthermore, the laboratory methods to detect imprinting defects on DNA level differed remarkably due to the lack of standardized methods and sets of imprinted loci and CpGs in the past.

Nevertheless, the major reason for the considerable differences between some studies is caused by the mode of ascertainment. In fact, numerous studies on the frequency of ImpDis in ART-conceived cohorts had been carried out, but only some of them were based on complete ART registries whereas the majority comprised data of voluntary registries for AS or BWS (20). Among the latter, only for BWS sufficient data to draw conclusions are available, whereas reports on ART in other IDs are mainly based on small cohorts or single cases (Table 7.1).

In fact, the influence of ART-associated treatment on the fine-tuned balance of the expression of imprinted genes can explain the occurrence of epimutations. However, it does not explain the occurrence of genomic alterations like deletions which have been reported in AS patients born after ART. These might be linked to the generally increased risk for congenital anomalies in ART-conceived children (17). However, for BWS as the most frequently observed ImpDis in children born after ART CNVs have not yet been reported in context with ART, but nearly all these children carried a ICR2 LOM. Another hint toward an influence of ART on imprinting marks is the observation that the majority of the respective ImpDis patients show a hypomethylation (e.g., ICR2 LOM in BWS, ICR1 LOM in SRS, SNURF: TSS-DMR LOM in AS), indicating an impact of ART procedures (e.g., cell culture conditions) on the maintenance of methylation.

Epidemiological Studies Based on ART Registries

In two large epidemiological studies from Sweden and Denmark, the number of children with ImpDis corresponded to the expected number in the naturally conceived cohort (21,22). In the Danish registry comprising 6,052 IVF/ICSI children, no case of BWS, SRS or PWS or another ImpDis could be identified. From the data of Swedish 16,280 ART-conceived, no evidence for an increased risk for ImpDis was obvious (21), respectively. In a survey of 2492 children born after ART in the Republic of Ireland and Central England, Bowdin et al. (23) overviewed clinical data for 1524 individuals. Out of these, 174 were reported to have one or more phenotypic features of an ImpDis, and 47 could be examined clinically. Four patients exhibited a BWS phenotype, but only one could be confirmed molecularly. Another child was diagnosed as AS but did not carry a AS-related molecular alteration. Finally, Bowdin and colleagues estimated an absolute risk for ImpDis of less than 1%. Studies in phenotypically normal children born after ART indirectly confirmed these observations as they did not reveal any enhanced variability of DNA methylation imprints (24). In summary, epidemiological studies from ART registries do not show any indication for an increased risk for ImpDis.

Studies Based on Patients Registries

Angelman Syndrome

AS was the first ImpDis that has been observed in context with ART. In 2002, Cox et al. (17) reported on two AS patients with sporadic inmprinting defects conceived after ICSI. As this molecular alteration is relatively rare (∼3%) in AS (25), the authors discussed for the first time whether ICSI might increase the risk of imprinting defects. After the third report of an AS patients with epimutation (18), Ludwig et al. (26) published a case control study on the frequency of subfertility/ART-conceived children among 79 AS children (subfertility was defined as time to pregnancy (TPP) >2 years and/or infertility treatment). Sixteen of these (20%) had a history of subfertility. The relative risk for AS was highest in couples with infertility treatment (hormone treatment/ICSI), but generally an increased incidence was observed in subfertile couples. Among the 16 patients, four had an imprinting defect (20%). Ten patients (62.5%) carried a deletion, which represents the most frequent alteration in AS but is difficult to be explained as the result of subfertility.

The authors concluded that imprinting defects and subfertility might have a common cause, but that the superovulation rather than the ART procedure itself has an increased risk for an imprinting defect. This observation was supported by Doornbos et al. in 2007 (27) in a case control study aiming on the frequency of infertility treatment/ART in a Dutch cohort of AS children. Eight out of 63 AS families had fertility problems (12.6%), and a significant association was found for AS children born after ovulation induction by drugs (4.8% vs. 0.39% in the Duch population). Molecular testing was performed in three of these eight patients and confirmed the clinical diagnosis. The molecular subgroup could be defined as deletions in two of them.

Further groups also addressed the relationship between AS and ART, with different results and partly incomplete documentation. A Japanese study included 123 AS patients ascertained via pediatric hospitals (28). Two of them were conceived after ART, but this frequency was not different from the expected rate. Furthermore, none of these two patients exhibited an epimutation. A similar study from the UK surveyed the reproductive data of 75 AS families via regional genetic centers (29). Three out of them had a history of assisted conception, among them two with a deletion.

Beckwith-Wiedemann Syndrome

The first case of BWS in a cohort of 73 children born after IVF/ICSI was published in 2001 (30), and in the following years several studies from the United States, United Kingdom, and France reported an increased frequency of (approximately four- to sixfold) ART births in BWS registries (31–33). In a population-based survey from Australia, Halliday et al. (34) also found an increased frequency of ART in children with BWS and calculated the estimated risk of BWS in the Australian IVF population as ~1/4,000, or 9 times greater than in the general population.

Molecular studies support this link between BWS and ART. With the exception of one patient with a putative upd(11)pat (31), all BWS patients born after ART and a molecularly proven diagnosis (n = 87), a hypomethylation at the KCNQ1OT1 TSS-DMR (ICR2) in 11p15 was identified (Table 7.2). This finding differs remarkably from that in AS where deletions and UPDs were also detectable in patients born after ART. In fact, the ICR2 hypomethylation contributes to 50% of the (epi)mutations in BWS, but due to the meanwhile large number of reported BWS-ART cases the occurrence of other molecular modifications than the ICR2 epimutation would have been expected.

Thus, it can be postulated that the ICR2 might be prone to altered methylation, and this is confirmed by the observation that this imprinted locus is the most frequently altered DMR in MLID patients. In summary, there is an obvious association between ICR2 hypomethylation in BWS and ART, but the data about an association between MLID and ART in BWS are inconclusive (14,35–37).

Silver-Russell Syndrome

The molecularly (and clinically) opposite syndrome to BWS is the growth retardation disease SRS. Nearly all 11p15 alterations detectable in BWS are also present in SRS, but affect the other parental allele (Table 7.1). Chromosome 11p15 disturbances account for more than 40% of patients, a further 7%–10% cases show disturbances affecting chromosome 7 (upd(7) mat; CNVs and epimutations of *GRB10* and *MEST* in single cases).

Up to now, 16 patients with features reminiscent to SRS born after ART have been reported. However, some of the case descriptions have to be regarded with caution because of the clinical heterogeneity of the disease and the unspecifity of symptoms. Until recently, the clinical diagnosis was mainly based on the experience of the clinician, and a standardized clinical scoring system has become available just two years ago (38,39). As a result the association of ART and ICR1 LOM in at least three out of the 16 cases in the literature is questionable because in these cases the diagnosis was not confirmed molecularly.

Whereas the first reports on SRS children born after ART comprised single cases, there are two studies on the screen for epimutations and ART in SRS. In 2012, Hiura et al. (28) published the results from a survey to estimate the number of SRS individuals in pediatric hospitals from Japan. Five out of the 42 children were conceived by ART, and four of them exhibited an MLID. The authors concluded a nearly tenfold higher frequency of ART in their SRS population. Another exceptional finding in that study was that four of these five patients exhibited a MLID, including GOM of several loci. In fact, MLID data obtained from peripheral lymphocytes DNA normally comprise hypomethylation at imprinted loci, whereas hypermethylation has rarely been described for fibroblasts from SRS patient (4). The second study aiming on epimutations and ART in a larger SRS cohort was carried out by Poole et al. (2013), they identified three children born after ART in a cohort of 23 patients with molecularly proven diagnosis. None of these three patients exhibited a MLID, at least in lymphocytes.

The occurrence of a chromosome 7 alteration in context with ART has been reported only once: Kagami et al. (40) reported on a patient with an isolated hypermethylation of *MEST* which was also present in minor degree in the father. Thus it is unclear whether the aggravation of the methylation in the course of the father-child transmission was caused by the ART procedure itself or not.

Prader-Willi Syndrome

For PWS, an association between ART and its occurrence could not be demonstrated in different surveys. In a Japanese cohort (n = 261), the frequency of ART-conceived patients with PWS was not different from the expected rage (4/261; 1.5%) (28). A Dutch case-control survey via patient support groups confirmed this negative finding after correction for the increased fertility problems of the parents (27).

Further Imprinting Disorders

With the exception of TNDM, ART has not been reported so far in patients with one of the other ImpDis. The reasons probably are that these ImpDis are either rare or have just recently been discovered. There is only one report on a patient with TNDM received after ART (29), identified by a case-control study after contacting families with known TNDM in the UK. In that cohort, among 23 patients only one patient carried a upd(6)pat.

7.7 CONCLUSION

With the first reports on children with ImpDis born after ART treatment, it was postulated that there should be a causal link between the ART procedure and aberrant methylation. In fact, this hypothesis was corroborated by different studies in mammals (14,15), but epidemiological studies in ART cohorts did not confirm an increase of children with ImpDis (21,22,27). However, numerous surveys in patient registries for BWS indicate that there is a significant increase of patients with epimutations conceived by ART, and this also becomes apparent for SRS. For AS as the first reported ImpDis in ART, this correlation is unclear, because several patients carry genomic alterations which are difficult to explain by the ART procedure itself. Therefore, the question remains whether the ART methodology or the sub/infertility itself is the risk factor resulting in an increased risk for children with congenital ImpDis born after ART (16). However, a combination of both is conceivable: The occurrence of some ImpDis like AS might be attributable to the generally slightly increased risk for congenital disorders in children born after IvF/ICSI due to the parental sub/infertility and the causes behind them, and some imprinted loci might be prone to an alteration of methylation marks caused by the ART procedure, for example, the 11p15 loci.

Further studies are needed to explore the apparently increased ratio of ImpDis patients born after ART. The parallel and comprehensive testing of different imprinted loci even in different tissues to detect MLID might further help to discriminate molecular subgroups of ImpDis patients born after ART, and this might help to decipher the putative causal link between the procedures and aberrant methylation of imprinted loci.

REFERENCES

1. Cardarelli L, Sparago A, De Crescenzo A et al. Silver-Russell syndrome and Beckwith-Wiedemann syndrome phenotypes associated with 11p duplication in a single family. *Pediatr Dev Pathol.* 2010;13:326–30.

2. Riess A, Binder G, Ziegler J et al. First report on concordant monozygotic twins with Silver-Russell syndrome and ICR1 hypomethylation. *Eur J Med Genet.* 2016;59:1–4.

3. Soellner L, Begemann M, Mackay DJ et al. Recent advances in imprinting disorders. *Clin Genet.* 2017;91:3–13.

4. Azzi S, Blaise A, Steunou V et al. Complex tissue-specific epigenotypes in Russell-Silver syndrome associated with 11p15 ICR1 hypomethylation. *Hum Mutat.* 2014;35:1211–20.

5. Mackay DJ, Eggermann T, Buiting K et al. Multilocus methylation defects in imprinting disorders. *Biomol Concepts.* 2015;6:47–57.

6. Abi Habib W, Brioude F, Azzi S et al. 11p15 ICR1 partial deletions associated with IGF2/H19 DMR hypomethylation and Silver-Russell syndrome. *Hum Mutat.* 2017;38:105–111.

7. Mackay DJ, Callaway JL, Marks SM et al. Hypomethylation of multiple imprinted loci in individuals with transient neonatal diabetes is associated with mutations in ZFP57. *Nat Genet.* 2008;40:949–51.

8. Eggermann K, Bliek J, Brioude F et al. EMQN best practice guidelines for the molecular genetic testing and reporting of chromosome 11p15 imprinting disorders: Silver-Russell and Beckwith-Wiedemann syndrome. *Eur J Hum Genet.* 2016;24:1377–87.

9. Bens S, Kolarova J, Beygo J et al. Phenotypic spectrum and extent of DNA methylation defects associated with multilocus imprinting disturbances. *Epigenomics.* 2016;8:801–16.

10. Docherty LE, Rezwan FI, Poole RL et al. Mutations in NLRP5 are associated with reproductive wastage and multilocus imprinting disorders in humans. *Nat Commun.* 2015;6:8086.

11. Meyer E, Lim D, Pasha S et al. Germline mutation in NLRP2 (NALP2) in a familial imprinting disorder (Beckwith-Wiedemann syndrome). *PLoS Genet.* 2009;5:e1000423.

12. Soellner L, Begemann M, Degenhardt F et al. Maternal heterozygous NLRP7 variant results in recurrent reproductive failure and imprinting disturbances in the offspring. *Eur J Hum Genet.* 2017;25:924–929.

13. Tee L, Lim DH, Dias RP et al. Epimutation profiling in Beckwith-Wiedemann syndrome: Relationship with assisted reproductive technology. *Clin Epigenetics.* 2013;5:23.

14. Chen Z, Hagen DE, Elsik CG et al. Characterization of global loss of imprinting in fetal overgrowth syndrome induced by assisted reproduction. *Proc Natl Acad Sci USA.* 2015;112:4618–23.

15. de Waal E, Yamazaki Y, Ingale P et al. Primary epimutations introduced during intracytoplasmic sperm injection (ICSI) are corrected by germline-specific epigenetic reprogramming. *Proc Natl Acad Sci USA.* 2012;109:4163–8.

16. Buckett WM, Tan SL. Congenital abnormalities in children born after assisted reproductive techniques: How much is associated with the presence of infertility and how much with its treatment? *Fertil Steril.* 2005;84:1318–9.

17. Cox GF, Bürger J, Lip V et al. Intracytoplasmic sperm injection may increase the risk of imprinting defects. *Am J Hum Genet* 2002;71:162–4.

18. Ørstavik KH, Eiklid K, van der Hagen CB et al. Another case of imprinting defect in a girl with Angelman syndrome who was conceived by intracytoplasmic semen injection. *Am J Hum Genet.* 2003;72:218–9.

19. Svensson J, Björnståhl A, Ivarsson SA. Increased risk of Silver-Russell syndrome after *in vitro* fertilization? *Acta Paediatr.* 2005 Aug;94(8):1163–5.
20. Vermeiden JP, Bernardus RE. Are imprinting disorders more prevalent after human *in vitro* fertilization or intracytoplasmic sperm injection? *Fertil Steril.* 2013;99:642–51.
21. Källén B, Finnström O, Lindam A et al. Congenital malformations in infants born after *in vitro* fertilization in Sweden. *Birth Defects Res A Clin Mol Teratol.* 2010;88:137–43.
22. Lidegaard Ø, Pinborg A, Andersen AN. Imprinting disorders after assisted reproductive technologies. *Curr Opin Obstet Gynecol.* 2006;18:293–6.
23. Bowdin S, Allen C, Kirby G et al. A survey of assisted reproductive technology births and imprinting disorders. *Hum Reprod.* 2007;22:3237–40.
24. Tierling S, Souren NY, Gries J et al. Assisted reproductive technologies do not enhance the variability of DNA methylation imprints in human. *J Med Genet.* 2010;47:371–6.
25. Buiting K, Clayton-Smith J, Driscoll DJ et al. Clinical utility gene card for: Angelman syndrome. *Eur J Hum Genet.* 2015;23(2), doi: 10.1038/ejhg.2014.93.
26. Ludwig M, Katalinic A, Gross S et al. Increased prevalence of imprinting defects in patients with Angelman syndrome born to subfertile couples. *J Med Genet.* 2005;42:289–91.
27. Doornbos ME, Maas SM, McDonnell J et al. Infertility, assisted reproduction technologies and imprinting disturbances: A Dutch study. *Hum Reprod.* 2007;22:2476–80.
28. Hiura H, Okae H, Miyauchi N et al. Characterization of DNA methylation errors in patients with imprinting disorders conceived by assisted reproduction technologies. *Hum Reprod.* 2012;27:2541–832.
29. Sutcliffe AG, Peters CJ, Bowdin S et al. Assisted reproductive therapies and imprinting disorders—A preliminary British survey. *Hum Reprod.* 2006;21:1009–11.
30. Olivennes F, Mannaerts B, Struijs M et al. Perinatal outcome of pregnancy after GnRH antagonist (ganirelix) treatment during ovarian stimulation for conventional IVF or ICSI: A preliminary report. *Hum Reprod.* 2001;16:1588–91.
31. DeBaun MR, Niemitz EL, Feinberg AP. Association of *in vitro* fertilization with Beckwith-Wiedemann syndrome and epigenetic alterations of LIT1 and H19. *Am J Hum Genet.* 2003;72:156–60.
32. Maher ER, Brueton LA, Bowdin SC et al. Beckwith-Wiedemann syndrome and assisted reproduction technology (ART). *J Med Genet.* 2003;40:62–4.
33. Gicquel C, Gaston V, Mandelbaum J et al. *In vitro* fertilization may increase the risk of Beckwith-Wiedemann syndrome related to the abnormal imprinting of the KCN1OT gene. *Am J Hum Genet.* 2003;72:1338–41.
34. Halliday J, Oke K, Breheny S et al. Beckwith-Wiedemann syndrome and IVF: A case-control study. *Am J Hum Genet.* 2004;75:526–8.
35. Rossignol S, Steunou V, Chalas C et al. The epigenetic imprinting defect of patients with Beckwith-Wiedemann syndrome born after assisted reproductive technology is not restricted to the 11p15 region. *J Med Genet.* 2006;43:902–7.
36. Lim D, Bowdin SC, Tee L et al. Clinical and molecular genetic features of Beckwith-Wiedemann syndrome associated with assisted reproductive technologies. *Hum Reprod.* 2009 Mar;24(3):741–7.
37. Poole RL, Docherty LE, Al Sayegh A et al. International clinical imprinting consortium. Targeted methylation testing of a patient cohort broadens the epigenetic and clinical description of imprinting disorders. *Am J Med Genet A.* 2013;161A:2174–82.

38. Azzi S, Salem J, Thibaud N et al. A prospective study validating a clinical scoring system and demonstrating phenotypical-genotypical correlations in Silver-Russell syndrome. *J Med Genet*. 2015;52:446–53.
39. Wakeling EL, Brioude F, Lokulo-Sodipe O et al. Diagnosis and management of Silver-Russell syndrome: First international consensus statement. *Nat Rev Endocrinol*. 2017;13:105–124.
40. Kagami M, Nagai T, Fukami M et al. Silver-Russell syndrome in a girl born after *in vitro* fertilization: Partial hypermethylation at the differentially methylated region of PEG1/MEST. *J Assist Reprod Genet*. 2007;24:131–6.
41. Chang AS, Moley KH, Wangler M et al. Association between Beckwith-Wiedemann syndrome and assisted reproductive technology: A case series of 19 patients. *Fertil Steril*. 2005;83:349–54.
42. Tenorio J, Romanelli V, Martin-Trujillo A et al. Clinical and molecular analyses of Beckwith-Wiedemann syndrome: Comparison between spontaneous conception and assisted reproduction techniques. *Am J Med Genet A*. 2016;170:2740–9.
43. Bliek J, Terhal P, van den Bogaard MJ et al. Hypomethylation of the H19 gene causes not only Silver-Russell syndrome (SRS) but also isolated asymmetry or an SRS-like phenotype. *Am J Hum Genet*. 2006;78:604–14.
44. Galli-Tsinopoulou A, Emmanouilidou E, Karagianni P et al. A female infant with Silver Russell syndrome, mesocardia, and enlargement of the clitoris. *Hormones (Athens)*. 2008;7:77–81.
45. Douzgou S, Mingarelli R, Tarani L et al. Silver-Russell syndrome following *in vitro* fertilization. *Pediatr Dev Pathol*. 2008;11:329–31.
46. Chopra M, Amor DJ, Sutton L et al. Russell-Silver syndrome due to paternal H19/IGF2 hypomethylation in a patient conceived using intracytoplasmic sperm injection. *Reprod Biomed Online*. 2010;20:843–7.
47. Cocchi G, Marsico C, Cosentino A et al. Silver-Russell syndrome due to paternal H19/IGF2 hypomethylation in a twin girl born after *in vitro* fertilization. *Am J Med Genet A*. 2013;161A:2652–5.

CHAPTER 8

Epigenetics and Assisted Reproduction Experimental Studies

Sperm Epigenome

Joan Blanco and Cristina Camprubí

CONTENTS

8.1 GENERAL OVERVIEW

Infertility is a common disease that affects between 8% and 12% of the couples worldwide, although with significant differences between high- and low-income countries (1). This disorder has been associated with a wide number of causes. Nevertheless, between 15% and 30% of the individuals asking for infertility, the origin remains classified as idiopathic (2). Since epigenetics plays a significant role in human germline development (Chapter 3), epigenetic alterations in gametes have been proposed to explain some idiopathic cases (3). Therefore, one explanation to the increased incidence of epigenetics disorders in ART (Chapter 6) has been related to conception using gametes of infertile couples that may have an elevated risk of epigenetic variations.

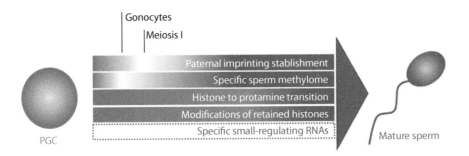

FIGURE 8.1 Progression of epigenetic changes along spermatogenesis. The paternal imprinting and specific sperm methylome stablishment, histone to protamine transition and modifications of retained histones occur at different stages along the formation of mature sperm from primordial germ cell (PGCs). RNA cargo is also represented but not as a dynamic process.

Although men and women contributed equally to human infertility (4), the intrinsic characteristics of oogenesis (related to sample obtainment, sample size, and epigenetics reprograming) have limited the number of studies addressing this topic in women. On the contrary, since the epigenome is fully reprogrammed in the mature sperm, and the number of cells available for the analysis is unlimited in most samples, studies in the field of infertility and epigenetics has been mainly focused on the male side.

As in all specialized cells in which the epigenome confers their specific function and genome mark of identity, the sperm epigenome consists of orchestrated factors playing together to guarantee sperm functions. Several studies have suggested that the sperm epigenome mirrors the correctness of the processes occurring during spermatogenesis and plays important roles in the developing embryo. Accordingly, several molecular factors have been involved in the epigenetic signature of sperm cells (Figure 8.1), although its specific function is still under debate.

In this chapter, we have reviewed the association between variations of the sperm epigenome and male infertility, with a particular emphasis in DNA methylation, nucleosome retention and chromatin protamination. The association between RNA cargo and male infertility is extensively developed in Chapter 9.

8.2 SPERM DNA METHYLATION

The sperm methylome is the result of the waves of genome-wide DNA reprogramming during the differentiation of primordial germ cells (PGCs) into spermatozoa (Chapter 4). Large-scale DNA methylation studies in human sperm from fertile individuals have revealed that the methylation profile of the sperm cell is highly polarized toward hypomethylation, with distinct functions of hypo- versus hypermethylated loci (5,6). Hypomethylated gene promoters are associated with spermatogenesis and early-embryo development processes (5–8). Moreover, sequences of repetitive DNA (ALU, SINES, LINES, α-SAT) appear to be methylated in spermatozoa, probably to prevent retrotransposition activity (7). Overall, authors have hypothesized that these features represent a footprint of spermatogenetic events, and are designed to ensure the first steps of the embryo developmental program. Accordingly, it seems plausible that abnormalities in the sperm methylome (probably in combination with histone-retention variations) may affect sperm quality leading to male infertility.

The study of the influence of sperm methylome over male infertility has been performed at two complementary levels. At the genome-wide level, variations have been associated with low sperm count (9,10), low sperm motility (11) abnormal chromatin sperm packaging (12) decreased fecundity (13) and poor embryo quality (14). The reason why broad differences of the sperm methylation affect male fertility probably relies on the uncovering of genes playing a significant role in spermatogenesis and embryogenesis. In this way, several studies have identified a relationship between male infertility and aberrant sperm-DNA methylation in specific loci: Imprinted genes (15); spermatogenesis-critical genes (9,16,17); ALU regions of repetitive DNA (18,19); and even genes unrelated to spermatogenesis (9,20).

Concerning the origin of these anomalies, we know that the epigenome is subject to alterations caused by intrinsic and extrinsic factors (Chapter 6). Variations in the DNA sequence of factors involved in the methylation of DNA during spermatogenesis have been associated with sperm methylome alterations. For instance, some authors have reported *DNMT3A* and *DNMT3L* variations in infertile patients with sperm DNA methylation anomalies at imprinted loci (21). A significant number of authors have focused their research in determining the influence on the availability of methyl groups provided by the folate metabolism. A key factor of this process is methylenetetrahydrofolate reductase (MTHFR). *MTHFR* 677C > T polymorphism has been associated with male infertility, although with controversial results. A recent meta-analysis (22) have suggested that this *MTHFR* polymorphism is associated with male infertility, except in cases of oligozoospermia. Other factors involved in sperm DNA methylations, such as the specific factor CCCTC-binding factor-like protein (CTCFL/BORIS) has been discarded (23,24). In any case, since the sperm methylome is the result of a complex machinery that involved the participation of a great number of molecules, the uncovering of the genetic factors involved in the occurrence of variations will require well-designed and high-quality studies using throughput methodologies.

Paternal age could be another factor that increase the possibility of alterations. Actually, the negative influence of age on the testicular function and seminogram is well documented (25). Some authors have found a widespread increase of sperm DNA methylation with age (26). This age effect over sperm methylation could uncover the methylation marks of groups of genes associated with fertility. For instance, in semen samples collected in the range of 9–19 years apart, it has been described a set of genes with significant changes over time (27). In this sense, Camprubí et al. (2016) supports the association between advanced age and sperm *RPS6KA2* hypermethylation (9). This gene encodes a member of the ribosomal S6 kinase (RSK) family of serine/threonine kinases implicated in controlling cell growth. Actually, the influence of age over DNA methylation goes beyond male fertility. It has been described that DNA from blood of old individuals is more heterogeneous and hypomethylated in comparison with newborn DNA (28). Moreover, premature aging diseases has been also related with variations in blood DNA methylation at specific loci (29).

Differences of sperm DNA methylation levels has also been related with obesity. Specifically, it has been described subtle sperm DNA methylation differences at specific CpG of imprinting loci in overweight/obese men (30). More impact results have been also recently described comparing sperm DNA methylation at a genome-wide level between lean and obese men, and between samples of obese men before and after gastric bypass surgery (31). Authors found methylation differences at more 1500 genes suggesting certain "hotspots" for methylation variations in the genome associated with changes in nutritional intake (31).

Beyond diet, some environmental factors such as Bisphenol-A have been related to differences in sperm DNA methylation (32) or hidroxymethylation (33). Persistent organic pollutants have been related with global sperm DNA hypomethylation (34). Finally, early life chemotherapy exposure has been also related with adult sperm epimutations supporting that exposure can promote epigenetic alterations that persist in later life (35). On this subject, we would like to remark the fact that the sperm is a easily obtainable cell type, which is repeatedly exposed to environment during its development, and with a well-known methylation pattern (6). These features makes the spermatozoa an ideal cell type to investigate the relationship between environmental factors and DNA methylation.

Concerning the study of the impact of sperm DNA methylation variations over ART outcome, there are controversial results. Some authors have associated the presence of sperm DNA methylation variations and low pregnancy rate, although other parameters such as fertilization rate and embryo quality were unaffected (36). On the contrary, other authors have not found any genome-wide effect of distinctive sperm DNA methylation on ART outcome (9). Recently, Denomme et al. (2017) have described sperm DNA methylation differences at retained histone CpG island between good and poor blastocyst development groups (37). In any case, an important consideration of all these studies is that sample size is relatively small; therefore, dataset is still limited to provide definite conclusions.

Besides the influence of sperm DNA methylation variation on embryo development, another question is still to be answered: Could germline DNA methylation variation be transmitted over generations? The detection of coding regions resistant to reprogramming (DNA methylation) in human primordial germ cells (PGCs) suggests the possibility of epigenetic inheritance (38). Recently, we found 97 genes annotated to regions described resistant to reprogramming in PGCs that keep a hypermethylated status in spermatozoa (6). Most of these regions are part of the gene body, suggesting a role of these regions resistant to reprogramming in the regulation of transcription and splicing mechanisms (39). Moreover, resistant reprogramming regions are particularly enriched in genes associated with behavior and metabolic disorders that appear during adult life (6). These results argue in favor of these genes as strong candidates for sperm transgenerational epigenetic inheritance. Considering these data, if sperm DNA methylation variations affect resistant reprogramming regions, we could not discard the onset of disorders in the adult life instead on a detrimental effect in the first steps of embryo development.

8.3 SPERM CHROMATIN

During the postmeiotic differentiation of round spermatids into spermatozoa, chromatin is extensively remodeled resulting in nucleoprotamine (85%) and nucleohistone (15%) conferring a distinctive pattern of chromatin conformations (40). This process has a protective role and has been also associated with gene regulation at specific loci. Protection is achieved by the substitution of histones by protamines, which are basic proteins allowing the establishment of highly ordered and compacted toroid-chromatin structures. Residual nucleosomes are programmatically retained at regulatory sequences of loci involved in embryo development.

Histone Retention and Modifications

As some authors suggested long ago (40), histones are programmatically retained in mature human sperm in gene regulatory regions (41) including the promoters of developmental genes, microRNA genes, and imprinted loci (8). Moreover, as it happens in somatic cells, retained histones carry multiple post-translational modifications with both activating and silencing marks (Chapter 2). This suggests that histones in these selected regions are able to provide some degree of retained regulatory competence through histone tail modifications; that is, some regions of the sperm genome would have a certain epigenetic control of gene expression after fertilization (8,42). Actually, although sperm protamines are replaced by histones provided by the oocyte, it has been shown in mice embryos that sperm retained histones are unaffected by this process, and remain associated with the paternal genome in the early embryo (43).

A great diversity of post-translational histone modifications has been observed in human sperm (44) including activating and repressive marks (8,45). The activating H3K4me2 and H3K4me3 marks have been associated with promoters of genes involved in spermatogenesis, cell cycle and cell metabolism. These promoters are depleted of the repressive H3K27me3 mark, which in turn are enriched at developmental promoters that are repressed in early embryos. Moreover, promoters for genes encoding transcription factors important for embryonic development and morphogenesis have activating (H3K4me3) and repressive (H3K27me3) marks known as "bivalent domains." This bivalent marking leads to transcriptionally permissive and restrictive chromatin configurations, which has been associated with activation or repression of genes participating in the embryo development program (46). Besides, enrichment of H4K12ac (activating mark) at CTCF binding sites, and in the promoters of genes involved in embryo developmental has been observed in sperm retained histones (47). In addition to modifications such as lysine methylation and acetylation, examples of crotonylation, oxidation, phosphorylation, and arginine methylation have also been observed in human sperm (44).

Although the molecular basis for the programmatically histone retention is not fully understood (48) the overall mechanism of retention appears to be consistent among individuals leading to a similar sperm histone profile among samples (44). Taking all these results together, post-translationally modified histones may reflect spermatogenesis events and could facilitate gene expression in the following generation. Accordingly, it appears reasonable to believe that alterations in these processes could affect the sperm epigenome resulting in an inappropriate transfer of epigenetic information to the oocyte leading to infertility. Indeed, some studies have implicated aberrant histone tail modifications in the mature sperm with various forms of male infertility (Table 8.1).

Concerning the origin of defective sperm histone localization and modifications in infertile patients, it has been associated with deficient expression of JMJD1A and JMJD2A histone demethylases (52,53). Moreover, some authors have found in patients with defective histone retentions, variations in the expression of Piwi (Hiwi) proteins (involved in the inactivation of transposable elements) (54), or genetic defects of *DPY19L2* gene (required for sperm head elongation and acrosome formation during spermatogenesis) (55). Nevertheless, in these particular cases, we unknown whether these anomalies are the cause or the consequences of the histone alterations.

The fact that sperm histone modifications are transmitted to the embryo and are resistant to protein oocyte replacement, argues in favor of an effect beyond fertilization. Accordingly,

TABLE 8.1 Studies Reporting an Association between Altered Sperm Histone Tail Modifications and Male Infertility

Reference	Infertility Phenotype	Histone Tail Modifications
Hammoud et al. (49)	• Poor embryogenesis • Abnormal semen parameters/ altered protamination	• Random histone retention • Reduction of H3K4me and H3K27me at developmental promoters and imprinted genes
Steilmann et al. (50)	Impaired spermatogenesis	Changes of the distribution pattern of H3K9ac
La Spina et al. (51)	Poor motile fractions	Alteration of histone methylations

altered histone retention may result in abnormal reprogramming of the paternal pronucleus compromising embryo viability. Nevertheless, the clinical implications of the histone marks variations in infertile men are still under debate, and there is a need for future studies addressing this topic. It could have an effect if it is considered that DNA methylation and histone modifications are complementary mechanisms, and changes in DNA methylation may result in a clinical effect (36,37). Therefore, it is plausible to suggest that differences in DNA methylation might be coupled to abnormalities at sperm histones. This would compromise the epigenetic information provided by the sperm that would result in male infertility.

Sperm Protamination

During the transition from spermatids to spermatozoa, histones are mostly replaced by protamine 1 (P1) and protamine 2 (P2). This protein exchange result in a highly compacted nuclear structure that is essential to protect the paternal genome in transit from the male to the female reproductive track. Histone replacement depends on previous hyperacetylation of histone H4 mediated by CDY histone acetyltranferase. Moreover, the transcription factor cAMP-responsive element modulator (CREM) regulates gene expression of P1 and P2.

We know for a long time that altered sperm protamination leads to male infertility (56). Numerous studies have reported an association between abnormal P1/P2 ratio and male infertility. A recent meta-analysis have demonstrated a negative effect of the protamine ratio over a wide range of infertility phenotypes including patients with increased sperm DNA damage (57). Altered protamination have been associated with CDY gene deletions (58) and down-expression of CREM-mRNA (59) or CREM-protein (60).

Whether altered sperm protamination have a negative effect on ART outcome is still a matter of debate. Altered protamination has been associated with an altered sperm chromatin packaging and DNA damage (57), and hence, to the delivering of an altered sperm chromatin environment that could affect embryo viability. In this sense, although some authors have found a negligible effect on fertilization, embryo quality and pregnancy rate (61), there are several studies reporting an association between poor protamination and reduced fertilization rate (62–66), and embryo quality (62,67). However, in these studies sample size is small and therefore we have to be cautious to draw definitive conclusions.

Like histones, protamines exhibited post-translational modifications suggesting that these proteins could also play themselves a role after fertilization. For instance, in human sperm, protamines have been shown to be phosphorylated and acetylated (68,69). Moreover, they seemed to carry combinations of different modifications (69). But the fact that protamines are exchanged by histones provided by the oocyte (43) argues against an effect of post-translational protamines modifications beyond fertilization. In any case, the possibility that a protamine code plays a role in the early embryo is tempting and needs to be further investigated.

8.4 CONCLUDING REMARKS

In this chapter, we have provided strong evidence that variations of the sperm epigenome are clearly associated with human male infertility. Whether epigenome variations are the cause or the consequence of a compromised spermatogenesis is still unclear and represent an open area for future investigations. Concerning the consequences of sperm epigenome variations after fertilization, we would like to remark that there are no conclusive data indicating a significant effect over ART outcome. Moreover, the incidence of epigenetics alterations in ART derived conceptions is negligible compared to the estimated incidence from sperm studies. This discrepancy could have different explanations. First, it is important to note that most of the studies cited in this chapter analyze the whole population of spermatozoa of a given semen sample. Accordingly, results are expressed as an average value for the whole sperm population. Therefore, any epigenome variations do not indicate that all sperm within a sample are abnormal, but rather a significant proportion of the sperm population are. Second, the lack of a significant proportion of ART conceptus exhibiting sperm-epigenetic variations also suggests that reprogramming in the early embryo is highly efficient in the elimination and correction of the inherited paternal variation.

Some authors recommend the incorporation of sperm epigenome analysis as a male fertility marker that could be useful in the reproductive advice of human male infertility. Nevertheless, before the incorporation in clinics the following issues need to be addressed:

1. There are several techniques to interrogate the sperm epigenome (low and high coverage techniques) against different targets (DNA methylation, histones, protamines, and ncRNA). Several reports have demonstrated that when there is a sperm epigenome alteration in a particular target, there is also an affectation of the remaining molecules. Accordingly, there is a need for studies to prove which target and technique are more informative and are more adequate for their incorporation in clinics.

2. At the sperm level, there is a need for more case control studies in well-defined groups of patients (sample size, age matched, excluding genetic etiologies, controlling the influence of environmental factors and diet). These results would provide epigenetic biomarkers of infertility and the indications for this kind of analysis in sperm.

3. In the same way, the consequences of alterations must be analyzed after fertilization at the embryo, fetus, and live-births level. Consequences should only be uncovered through the implementation of randomized prospective studies using spermatozoa from patients exhibiting alterations compared with patients without alterations.

REFERENCES

1. Inhorn MC, Patrizio P. Infertility around the globe: New thinking on gender, reproductive technologies and global movements in the 21st century. *Hum Reprod Update.* 2014;21(4):411–26.
2. Practice Committee of the American Society for Reproductive Medicine. Effectiveness and treatment for unexplained infertility. *Fertil Steril.* 2006;86(5 Suppl.):S111–4.
3. Gunes S, Arslan MA, Hekim GNT, Asci R. The role of epigenetics in idiopathic male infertility. Vol. 33, *J Assist Reprod Genet.* 2016;33(5):553–69.
4. Dohle GR, Colpi GM, Hargreave TB et al. EAU guidelines on male infertility. *Eur Urol.* 2005;48:703–11.
5. Krausz C, Sandoval J, Sayols S et al. Novel insights into DNA Methylation features in Spermatozoa: Stability and peculiarities. *PLoS One.* 2012;7(10):e44479.
6. Camprubí C, Cigliano RA, Salas-Huetos A et al. What the human sperm methylome tells us. *Epigenomics.* 2017;9(10):1299–1315.
7. Molaro A, Hodges E, Fang F et al. Sperm methylation profiles reveal features of epigenetic inheritance and evolution in primates. *Cell.* 2011;146(6):1029–41.
8. Hammoud SS, Nix DA, Zhang H et al. Distinctive chromatin in human sperm packages genes for embryo development. *Nature.* 2009;460(7254):473–8.
9. Camprubí C, Salas-Huetos A, Aiese-Cigliano R et al. Spermatozoa from infertile patients exhibit differences of DNA methylation associated with spermatogenesis-related processes: An array-based analysis. *Reprod Biomed Online.* 2016;33(6):709–19.
10. Schütte B, El Hajj N, Kuhtz J et al. Broad DNA methylation changes of spermatogenesis, inflammation, and immune response-related genes in a subgroup of sperm samples for assisted reproduction. *Andrology.* 2013;1:822–9.
11. Pacheco SE, Houseman EA, Christensen BC et al. Integrative DNA methylation and gene expression analyses identify DNA packaging and epigenetic regulatory genes associated with low motility sperm. *PLoS One.* 2011;6(6):1–10.
12. Aston KI, Punj V, Liu L, Carrell DT. Genome-wide sperm deoxyribonucleic acid methylation is altered in some men with abnormal chromatin packaging or poor *in vitro* fertilization embryogenesis. *Fertil Steril.* 2012;97(2):285–292.
13. Jenkins TG, Aston KI, Meyer TD et al. Decreased fecundity and sperm DNA methylation patterns. *Fertil Steril.* 2016;105(1):51–57.
14. Aston KI, Uren PJ, Jenkins TG et al. Aberrant sperm DNA methylation predicts male fertility status and embryo quality. *Fertil Steril.* 2015; 104(6):1388–97.
15. Santi D, De Vincentis S, Magnani E, Spaggiari G. Impairment of sperm DNA methylation in male infertility: A meta-analytic study. *Andrology.* 2017;5(4):695–703.
16. Nanassy L, Carrell DT. Analysis of the methylation pattern of six gene promoters in sperm of men with abnormal protamination. *Asian J Androl.* 2011;13(2):342–6.
17. Navarro-Costa P, Nogueira P, Carvalho M et al. Incorrect DNA methylation of the DAZL promoter CpG island associates with defective human sperm. *Hum Reprod.* 2010;25(10):2647–54.
18. El Hajj N, Zechner U, Schneider E et al. Methylation status of imprinted genes and repetitive elements in sperm DNA from infertile males. *Sex Dev.* 2011;5(2):60–9.
19. Urdinguio RG, Bayón GF, Dmitrijeva M et al. Aberrant DNA methylation patterns of spermatozoa in men with unexplained infertility. *Hum Reprod.* 2015; 30(5):1014–28.

20. Houshdaran S, Cortessis VK, Siegmund K et al. Widespread epigenetic abnormalities suggest a broad DNA methylation erasure defect in abnormal human sperm. *PLoS One.* 2007;2(12):e1289.

21. Kobayashi H, Hiura H, John RM et al. DNA methylation errors at imprinted loci after assisted conception originate in the parental sperm. *Eur J Hum Genet.* 2009;17(12):1582–91.

22. Gong M, Dong W, He T et al. MTHFR 677C>T polymorphism increases the male infertility risk: A meta-analysis involving 26 studies. *PLoS One.* 2015;10(3):e0121147.

23. Poplinski A, Tüttelmann F, Kanber D et al. Idiopathic male infertility is strongly associated with aberrant methylation of MEST and IGF2/H19 ICR1. *Int J Androl.* 2010;33:642–9.

24. Camprubí C, Pladevall M, Grossmann M et al. Lack of association of MTHFR rs1801133 polymorphism and CTCFL mutations with sperm methylation errors in infertile patients. *J Assist Reprod Genet.* 2013;30(9):1125–31.

25. Eisenberg ML, Meldrum D. Effects of age on fertility and sexual function. *Fertil Steril.* 2017;107(2):301–4.

26. Jenkins TG, Aston KI, Cairns BR, Carrell DT. Paternal aging and associated intraindividual alterations of global sperm 5-methylcytosine and 5-hydroxymethylcytosine levels. *Fertil Steril.* 2013;100(4):945–51.

27. Jenkins TG, Aston KI, Pflueger C et al. Age-associated sperm DNA methylation alterations: Possible implications in offspring disease susceptibility. *PLoS Genet.* 2014;10(7):e1004458.

28. Heyn H, Li N, Ferreira HJ et al. Distinct DNA methylomes of newborns and centenarians. *Proc Natl Acad Sci.* 2012;109(26):10522–7.

29. Heyn H, Moran S, Esteller M. Aberrant DNA methylation profiles in the premature aging disorders Hutchinson-Gilford Progeria and Werner syndrome. *Epigenetics.* 2013;8(1):28–33.

30. Soubry A, Guo L, Huang Z et al. Obesity-related DNA methylation at imprinted genes in human sperm: Results from the TIEGER study. *Clin Epigenetics.* 2016;8(1):51.

31. Donkin I, Versteyhe S, Ingerslev LR et al. Obesity and bariatric surgery drive epigenetic variation of spermatozoa in humans. *Cell Metab.* 2016;23(2):369–78.

32. Miao M, Zhou X, Li Y et al. LINE-1 hypomethylation in spermatozoa is associated with Bisphenol A exposure. *Andrology.* 2014;2(1):138–44.

33. Zheng H, Zhou X, Li DK et al. Genome-wide alteration in DNA hydroxymethylation in the sperm from bisphenol A-exposed men. *PLoS One.* 2017;12(6):e0178535.

34. Consales C, Toft G, Leter G et al. Exposure to persistent organic pollutants and sperm DNA methylation changes in Arctic and European populations. *Environ Mol Mutagen.* 2016;57(3):200–9.

35. Shnorhavorian M, Schwartz SM, Stansfeld B et al. Differential DNA methylation regions in adult human sperm following adolescent chemotherapy: Potential for epigenetic inheritance. *PLoS One.* 2017;12(2):e0170085.

36. Benchaib M, Braun V, Ressnikof D et al. Influence of global sperm DNA methylation on IVF results. *Hum Reprod.* 2005;20(3):768–73.

37. Denomme MM, McCallie BR, Parks JC et al. Alterations in the sperm histone-retained epigenome are associated with unexplained male factor infertility and poor blastocyst development in donor oocyte IVF cycles. *Hum Reprod.* 2017;32(12):1–13.

38. Tang WWCWC, Dietmann S, Irie N et al. A unique gene regulatory network resets the human germline epigenome for development. *Cell.* 2015;161(6):1453–67.

39. Jones PA. Functions of DNA methylation: Islands, start sites, gene bodies and beyond. *Nat Rev Genet.* 2012;13(7):484–92.

40. Gatewood JM, Cook GR, Balhorn R et al. Sequence-specific packaging of DNA in human sperm chromatin. *Science*. 1987;236(4804):962–4.
41. Arpanahi A, Brinkworth M, Iles D et al. Endonuclease-sensitive regions of human spermatozoal chromatin are highly enriched in promoter and CTCF binding sequences. *Genome Res*. 2009;19(8):1338–49.
42. Arpanahi A, Brinkworth M, Iles D et al. Endonuclease-sensitive regions of human spermatozoal chromatin are highly enriched in promoter and CTCF binding sequences. *Genome Res*. 2009;19:1338–49.
43. Van Der Heijden GW, Ramos L, Baart EB et al. Sperm-derived histones contribute to zygotic chromatin in humans. *BMC Dev Biol*. 2008;8(1):34.
44. Luense LJ, Wang X, Schon SB et al. Comprehensive analysis of histone post-translational modifications in mouse and human male germ cells. *Epigenetics Chromatin*. 2016;9(1):24.
45. Brykczynska U, Hisano M, Erkek S et al. Repressive and active histone methylation mark distinct promoters in human and mouse spermatozoa. *Nat Struct Mol Biol*. 2010;17(6): 679–87.
46. Bernstein BE, Mikkelsen TS, Xie X et al. A bivalent chromatin structure marks key developmental genes in embryonic stem cells. *Cell*. 2006;125(2):315–26.
47. Paradowska AS, Miller D, Spiess AN et al. Genome wide identification of promoter binding sites for H4K12ac in human sperm and its relevance for early embryonic development. *Epigenetics*. 2012;7(9):1057–70.
48. Johnson GD, Lalancette C, Linnemann AK et al. The sperm nucleus: Chromatin, RNA, and the nuclear matrix. *Reproduction*. 2011;141(1):21–36.
49. Hammoud SS, Nix DA, Hammoud AO et al. Genome-wide analysis identifies changes in histone retention and epigenetic modifications at developmental and imprinted gene loci in the sperm of infertile men. *Hum Reprod*. 2011;26(9):2558–69.
50. Steilmann C, Paradowska A, Bartkuhn M et al. Presence of histone H3 acetylated at lysine 9 in male germ cells and its distribution pattern in the genome of human spermatozoa. *Reprod Fertil Dev*. 2011;23(8):997–1011.
51. La Spina FA, Romanato M, Brugo-Olmedo S et al. Heterogeneous distribution of histone methylation in mature human sperm. *J Assist Reprod Genet*. 2014;31(1):45–9.
52. Eelaminejad Z, Favaedi R, Sodeifi N et al. Deficient expression of JMJD1A histone demethylase in patients with round spermatid maturation arrest. *Reprod Biomed Online*. 2017;34(1):82–9.
53. Okada Y, Tateishi K, Zhang Y. Histone demethylase JHDM2A is involved in male infertility and obesity. *J Androl*. 2010;31(1):75–8.
54. Gou L-T, Kang J-Y, Dai P et al. Ubiquitination-deficient mutations in human Piwi cause male infertility by impairing histone-to-protamine exchange during Spermiogenesis. *Cell*. 2017;169(6):1090–1104.
55. Yassine S, Escoffier J, Martinez G et al. Dpy19l2-deficient globozoospermic sperm display altered genome packaging and DNA damage that compromises the initiation of embryo development. *Mol Hum Reprod*. 2015;21(2):169–85.
56. Balhorn R, Reed S, Tanphaichitr N. Aberrant protamine 1/protamine 2 ratios in sperm of infertile human males. *Experientia*. 1988;44(1):52–5.
57. Ni K, Spiess A-N, Schuppe H-C, Steger K. The impact of sperm protamine deficiency and sperm DNA damage on human male fertility: A systematic review and meta-analysis. *Andrology*. 2016;4(5):789–99.

58. Sonnack V, Failing K, Bergmann M, Steger K. Expression of hyperacetylated histone H4 during normal and impaired human spermatogenesis. *Andrologia*. 2002;34(6):384–90.

59. Steger K, Klonisch T, Gavenis K et al. Round spermatids show normal testis-specific H1t but reduced cAMP-responsive element modulator and transition protein 1 expression in men with round-spermatid maturation arrest. *J Androl*. 1999;20(6):747–54.

60. Weinbauer GF, Behr R, Bergmann M, Nieschlag E. Testicular cAMP responsive element modulator (CREM) protein is expressed in round spermatids but is absent or reduced in men with round spermatid maturation arrest. *Mol Hum Reprod*. 1998;4(1):9–15.

61. Hammadeh ME, Al-Hasani S, Stieber M et al. The effect of chromatin condensation (aniline blue staining) and morphology (strict criteria) of human spermatozoa on fertilization, cleavage, and pregnancy rates in an intracytoplasmic sperm injection programme. *Hum Reprod*. 1996;11(11):2468–71.

62. Depa-Martynow M, Kempisty B, Jagodziński PP et al. Impact of protamine transcripts and their proteins on the quality and fertilization ability of sperm and the development of preimplantation embryos. *Reprod Biol*. 2012;12(1):57–72.

63. Nasr-Esfahani MH, Salehi M, Razavi S et al. Effect of sperm DNA damage and sperm protamine deficiency on fertilization and embryo development post-ICSI. *Reprod Biomed Online*. 2005;11(2):198–205.

64. Esterhuizen AD, Franken DR, Lourens JG et al. Sperm chromatin packaging as an indicator of *in vitro* fertilization rates. *Hum Reprod*. 2000;15(3):657–61.

65. Iranpour FG. Impact of sperm chromatin evaluation on fertilization rate in intracytoplasmic sperm injection. *Adv Biomed Res*. 2014;3:229.

66. Nasr-Esfahani MH, Razavi S, Mozdarani H et al. Relationship between protamine deficiency with fertilization rate and incidence of sperm premature chromosomal condensation post-ICSI. *Andrologia*. 2004;36(3):95–100.

67. Marchiani S, Tamburrino L, Benini F et al. Chromatin protamination and catsper expression in spermatozoa predict clinical outcomes after assisted reproduction programs. *Sci Rep*. 2017;7(1):15122.

68. Brunner AM, Nanni P, Mansuy IM. Epigenetic marking of sperm by post-translational modification of histones and protamines. *Epigenetics Chromatin*. 2014;7(1):2.

69. Oliva R, Castillo J, Estanyol J, Ballescà J. Human sperm chromatin epigenetic potential: Genomics, proteomics, and male infertility. *Asian J Androl*. 2015;17(4):601.

CHAPTER 9

Epigenetic and Assisted Reproduction Experimental Studies

Sperm ncRNAs

Celia Corral-Vazquez and Ester Anton

CONTENTS

9.1 INTRODUCTION

Spermatozoa are highly differentiated cells that play an essential role in reproduction by providing the haploid paternal genome to the embryo. For a long time, this contribution was considered the only function of spermatozoa, but several studies have revealed that these cells encompass a wider range of implications at both pre-fertilization and post-fertilization levels.

Therefore, the biological relevance of sperm cells is not merely based on DNA, but also proteins and RNA. Although the scarce sperm RNA amount (about 200 times less than somatic cells) was either ignored or considered a mere residual pool from previous spermatogenic processes (1), recent findings have revealed that sperm RNAs include a functional and complex population of molecules, with a wide range of subtypes and roles. This cargo constitutes an interesting resource for basic and applied research in the field of male infertility (2,3).

Sperm RNAs comprise a coding fraction (mRNAs), but also a non-coding set of RNAs (non-coding RNAs or ncRNAs). This last group can be divided, depending on their length, into large non-coding RNA (lncRNA) and small non-coding RNA (sncRNA). It has been estimated that large RNAs (mRNAs and lncRNAs) constitute about 50 fg (femtograms) of the total sperm RNA fraction, and sncRNAs contribute with $\sim$0.3 fg (4). Although ncRNAs were initially considered as junk RNA, many biological functions have been recently described for these molecules, highlighting their involvement in gene expression regulation (5).

9.2 LONG NON-CODING RNA

Monocatenary ncRNAs with a length of >200 nucleotides (nt) are classified into the category of long non-coding RNAs. Most of these molecules are transcribed as mRNAs by RNA polymerase II, but they can also be generated by the processing of other kinds of transcripts. In contrast to sncRNAs, their functionality does not depend on their attachment to proteins (5).

The biological functions of lncRNAs mainly comprise several epigenetic regulation pathways, affecting either the transcription of single mRNAs or even whole chromosomes (6). Their regulatory role has been categorized into three different modes: *Competitor, recruiter/activator,* and *precursor* (5) (Figure 9.1). The *competitor mode* concerns the ability of these molecules to impede the function of DNA regulatory proteins (e.g., transcription factors) either by attaching to these proteins or by blocking their target DNA regions (5,7). The *recruiter/activator mode* is related to the enhancement of DNA epigenetic alterations, such as histone modifications (8) or DNA methylation (9,10). lncRNA can bind to certain epigenetic modifiers and activate or recruit them to their specific target sites. Finally, the *precursor mode* comprises lncRNA processing by RNases (e.g., DROSHA and DICER) in order to generate shorter RNAs involved in post-transcriptional gene regulation (11).

There are specific types of lncRNAs that are especially abundant in the sperm transcriptome. Some of these transcripts have been found to be associated with chromatin, known as Chromatin-associated RNAs (CARs). It has been suggested that CARs can influence genome architecture and regulate gene expression (1). Another kind of abundant lncRNAs are the snaRs (small-nuclear ILF3/NF30 associated RNAs), specifically *snaR-G1*, which is over 100 times more highly expressed in sperm in comparison with testes or somatic tissues. This transcript appears to be involved into the regulation of human chorionic gonadotrophin (*hCG1*) transcription (1).

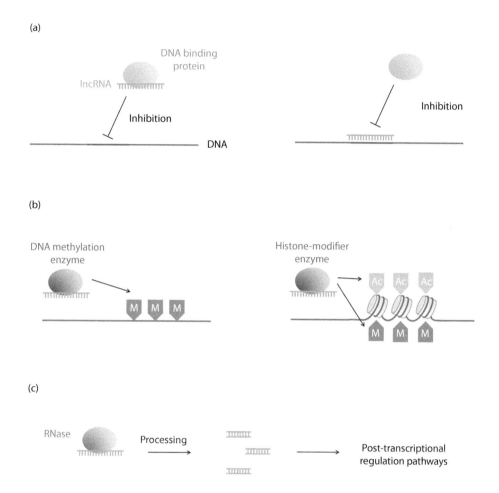

FIGURE 9.1   Molecular mechanisms of regulation associated to long non-coding RNAs (lncRNAs). (a) Competitor mechanism consists on the inhibition of gene expression by the attachment of lncRNAs to DNA binding proteins or to their target sequences. (b) Recruiter/activator mechanism refers to the activation of epigenetic modifiers and their recruitment to their specific target sites. (c) Precursor mechanism comprises the processing of lncRNAs by certain RNases into shorter RNAs that can be involved in further post-transcriptional regulation pathways.

9.3 SMALL NON-CODING RNA

The sncRNA family is composed of several categories of 20–300 nt transcripts. Although all of them share a strong regulatory role, they can be classified according to their size, biosynthesis pathway, type of associated proteins, and mechanism of action (1). Mainly, they divide into miRNAs, piRNAs, and endo-siRNAs (12). In addition, other classes of sncRNAs are also found in spermatozoa: Repetitive elements, transcription start sites (TSS)/promoter associated RNAs, small nuclear RNAs (snRNAs), small nucleolar RNAs (snoRNAs), mature-sperm-enriched tRNA-derived small RNAs (mse-tsRNAs), and YRNAs (13).

microRNA

miRNAs are monocatenary RNA molecules of approximately 22 nt in size. Their regulatory function is generally based on their complementary attachment to 3′ UTR regions of target mRNAs, consequently inhibiting their expression (14). Alternatively, miRNAs can bind to other genomic regions, such as promoters, and act as transcriptional regulators (15). A single miRNA can target multiple genes, and a single gene can be targeted by several miRNA. It is estimated that the expression of more than 60% of genes are regulated by miRNAs (14).

The synthesis of miRNAs starts in the nucleus with the transcription of RNA hairpins, named primary miRNAs (pri-miRNAs). This transcription is generally performed by polymerase II (16). The miRNA coding regions are generally isolated and widespread along the whole genome, although some of them are clustered together. These clusters are transcribed as single long precursors and then processed into individual miRNAs (17). The hairpin structures are cleaved by the microprocessor complex, which comprises an RNase III-type nuclease (DROSHA) and DiGeorge Syndrome Critical Region 8 (DGCR8). The generated intermediate precursors (pre-miRNAs) are transported to the cytoplasm through nuclear pores by Exportin-5. The RNase III endonuclease, DICER, processes these precursors and creates ∼22 base pairs duplex (miRNA:miRNA*). Afterward, the functionally mature monocatenary miRNAs are originated (14). In most cases, only one strand of the miRNA:miRNA* duplex remains functional while the other one is degraded (the miRNA* strand). Nevertheless, in some cases both of them can become functional (18). For example, it has been discovered that both strands remain functional in most miRNA duplex precursors of certain tissues, including testis (19). Mature miRNA molecules are attached to Argonaute (Ago) and TNRC6 (trinucleotide repeat-containing 6) proteins, forming the ribonucleoprotein miRNA-induced silencing complex (miRISC) (20) (Figure 9.2).

Several studies have revealed that hundreds of different miRNAs are expressed in mammalian testes. Also, nearly 40% of them are expressed differentially in comparison with somatic tissues (19,21). Many of the coding sequences of these prominently testicular miRNAs are placed on the X chromosome (19). Besides, the characterization of human sperm miRNAs has revealed the existence of a specific expression profile in fertile males. A study performed in 10 fertile individuals showed a panel of 221 miRNAs that were present in all their sperm samples. The regulatory pathways of these ncRNAs were found to be involved in biological processes related to spermatogenesis and embryogenesis (22). Another characterization of sperm ncRNA of fertile men revealed the presence of 35

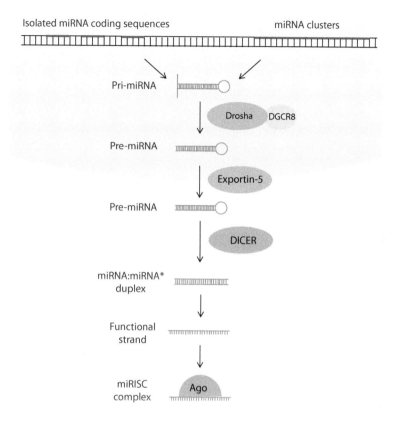

FIGURE 9.2   Biosynthesis pathway of microRNAs (miRNAs). Primary miRNAs (pri-miRNAs) are transcribed from clustered or isolated sequences and processed into pre-miRNA precursors. They are transported to the cytoplasm and processed by DICER into miRNA duplex. The functional strands of the duplex molecules are attached to Ago proteins and form the miRNA-induced silencing complex (miRISC).

enriched miRNAs that were involved in embryo development and cell growth processes (13). Regarding other expression studies performed in fertile men, it has been found that several miRNAs, such as hsa-miR-34b-3p, hsa-miR-375, and hsa-miR-191-5p, are overexpressed in human sperm cells (22,23).

piRNA

piRNAs are 24–30 nt monocatenary RNAs. They are attached to PIWI proteins, which are exclusive of germline cells and are classified into three main groups in mice: PIWIL1/MIWI, PIWIL2/MILI, and PIWIL4/MIWI2 (24). These molecules have been found to be the most abundant ncRNA in both human and mice sperm transcriptomes (12,25).

Biological functions of piRNAs are focused around the regulation of retrotransposons, serving as a protection mechanism against genome modifications produced by these transposable elements (24). In sperm cells, *LINE1* (long interspersed nuclear elements 1) constitute the most frequently regulated retrotransposons by piRNAs (25). The regulation of transposable elements can be performed either post-transcriptionally or by epigenetic modifications. Post-transcriptional silencing is caused by piRNA attachment to complementary retrotransposon sequences, causing their degradation. Besides this silencer role, piRNAs have also been suggested to participate in the regulation of *de novo* methylation in embryos and prospermatogonias. However, this last mechanism still needs to be completely characterized (24).

piRNAs are codified in several clusters, widespread in different chromosomal regions. The size of these clusters can vary from a few nucleotides to hundreds of kilobases (26). Each cluster comprises several non-overlapping piRNA sequences. Two models of piRNA biosynthesis have been established from studies in mice cells: The *primary* pathway and the *secondary* mechanism ("ping-pong") (24) (Figure 9.3). It has been suggested that both models could be extrapolated to human piRNA biosynthesis (12).

The *primary* processing model starts with the transcription of a precursor RNA from cluster sequences. Unlike miRNAs, this molecule does not adopt a hairpin structure and, therefore, does not require DICER intervention. Instead, it is processed by nucleases that generate a primary piRNA. This molecule usually presents a 5′ ending with a phosphate group (PIWI binding site), and a 3′ ending with an OH group and a 2′-OH methylation. The size of these primary piRNAs depends on the footprint of the associated PIWI proteins: ∼26 nucleotides for MILI, ∼28 nucleotides for MIWI2, and 29–30 nucleotides for MIWI (24).

The *secondary* "ping-pong" cycle concerns the synthesis of piRNAs from transcripts with a primary piRNA complementary sequence. It has been observed that a significant fraction of piRNAs display a 5′ overlapping region of 10 nt. Some of them are enriched for uridine at the 5′ end while their complementary piRNAs are enriched for adenine at position 10. These coinciding structures are the outcome of the occurrence of the *secondary* mechanism. When primary piRNAs bind to their complementary RNAs, PIWI proteins cleave the target transcripts at the adenine located at position 10. This way, they generate a piRNA precursor with a 5′ uridine. The 3′ end is processed, and a new, mature secondary piRNA is then attached to MIWI2, becoming functional. This mechanism is closely related to the regulation of retrotransposons, since they mainly comprise target sequences of primary piRNAs (24).

endo-siRNA

The endo-siRNAs are 22 nt RNA molecules. Originally, they were discovered in yeast, plants, and *C. elegans*, but more recently were also identified in mammal cells (27). Even though these sncRNAs are found in all kinds of tissues (14), studies performed in mice

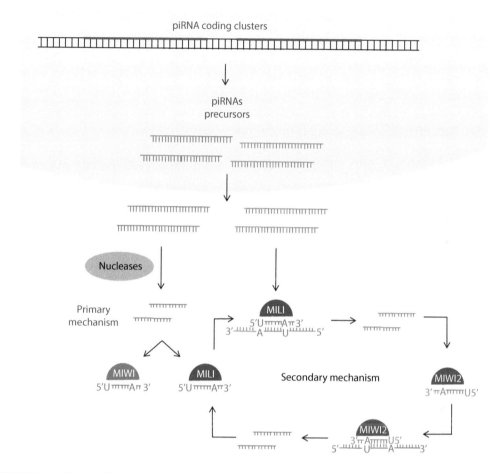

FIGURE 9.3   Biosynthesis of piRNAs. Molecules of piRNA precursors are transcribed from piRNA coding clusters and exported to cytoplasm. The primary biosynthesis mechanism comprises the processing of these precursors into primary piRNAs that bind to PIWI proteins. In the secondary "ping-pong" mechanism, primary piRNAs are attached to complementary sequences and process them into new secondary piRNAs.

have revealed higher expression levels in male germ cells. Specifically, 73 testicular endo-siRNAs have been characterized by RNA-seq, whose target sequences mainly correspond to mRNAs (92%), but also ncRNAs (4%), pseudogenes (3%), and retrotransposons (1%) (27).

The regulatory role of endo-siRNAs is similar to the gene silencing pathway of miRNAs, although they differ in the biosynthetic process. Endo-siRNAs derive from a double-stranded RNA (dsRNA) precursor. Two types of precursors can be generated: *Trans*-nat-dsRNAs (if each strand comes from a different loci) or *cis*-nat-dsRNA (if both strands come from bidirectional transcription of a single locus) (27). Precursor dsRNAs are transported to cytoplasm and processed by DICER, without the intervention of DROSHA-DGCR8. One of the strands will bind to an Ago protein and generate the RNA-induced silencing complex (RISC) (Figure 9.4).

The post-transcriptional gene regulatory function of endo-siRNAs is based on their attachment to 3′ UTR regions of the target mRNAs (27). These transcripts can be either silenced or degraded by the RISC complex, depending on the complementarity degree of endo-siRNA and mRNA sequences (14).

Regarding their biological implication in sperm cells, a possible extra role of endo-siRNAs in transcriptional regulation has been detected. It has been discovered that these sncRNAs guide epigenetic elements, such as histone methyltransferases, and promote the modification of chromatin conformation (27). Additionally, some studies suggest that endo-siRNAs are necessary in post-fertilization processes for the correct development of preimplantational embryos (28).

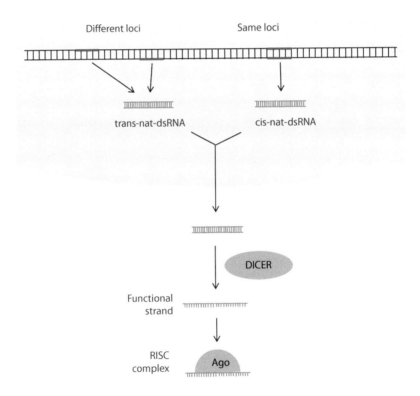

FIGURE 9.4 Double-stranded endo-siRNA precursors are originated and transported to the cytoplasm. They are processed by DICER and the functional strands bind to Ago proteins and form the RNA-induced silencing complex (RISC).

9.4 SPERM ncRNAs AND THEIR IMPLICATION DURING SPERMATOGENESIS

Spermatogenesis is a complex process that leads spermatogonia to proliferate, undertake meiosis, and differentiate into spermatozoa. Therefore, this process is composed by three main stages: Mitotic, meiotic, and postmeiotic (3). Most major cellular changes that occur during spermatogenesis take place postmeiotically. In this last stage, round spermatids undergo structural modifications: Cytoplasm elimination and formation of acrosome and flagellum. Within the nucleus, most of the histones are replaced by protamines, and chromatin is condensed in a highly packaged structure (29,30). Transcriptional activity continues from the beginning of spermatogenesis until the formation of round spermatids. At this step, transcription is arrested, coinciding with acrosome formation and chromatin repackaging (31). During the transcriptionally active phase, RNA synthesis significantly increases in two transcriptional waves: One of them takes place during the premeiotic cell stage (spermatogonia), while the other one occurs at the intermediate point between pachytene and the round spermatid stage. During these highly regulated waves, specific transcripts needed for the correct development of each stage are generated (32). Besides coding RNAs, sperm transcripts involved in spermatogenesis development also comprise many ncRNAs (1). In fact, several pathways involved in spermatogenesis regulation have been attributed to different spermatic lncRNAs, miRNAs, piRNAs, and endo-siRNAs.

Several lncRNAs have been characterized in male germ cells, with a potential influence over the whole spermatogenetic process. Nevertheless, only a few of them have been actually detected in differentiated spermatozoa. Some examples are DMR (DMRT1 related gene), which targets the mRNAs of *DMRT1* (a transcription factor involved in germ cell development and related to spermatogonia differentiation regulation), and *Spga-lncRNA1/2*, which seems to play a role in spermatogonia pluripotency preservation. Although they have been detected in sperm cells, both are initially expressed in spermatogonia. Additionally, some other lncRNAs have been detected in pachytene spermatocytes, like *MRHL* (meiotic recombination hot spot locus) and *TSX* (testis-specific X-linked), involved in meiosis regulation (5).

Regarding sncRNAs, the involvement of miRNAs in the regulation of human spermatogenesis has begun to be characterized. Although miRNA transcription is quite abundant throughout the whole process, transcriptional waves also influence their biosynthesis. During the first wave, many miRNAs involved in the preservation of the spermatogonia niche are produced. Some examples discovered in mice are miR-20, miR-21, miR-34c, miR-106a, mir-135a, miR-146a, miR-182, miR-183 miR-17-92 cluster, miR-221, and miR-222 (32,33). Other miRNAs take an opposite part in this regulation and promote spermatogonia differentiation, like let-7 family or miR-383 (32,34). In the second transcriptional wave, miRNAs that regulate a wide range of cellular mechanisms are produced. These processes include massive apoptosis (miR-449 cluster and miR-34b/c), chromatin rearrangement, sperm maturation (miR-18 and miR-214), or the transcription of transition proteins and protamine genes (miR-469 and miR-122a) (32,33).

As well as gene silencing, retrotransposon control in germ cells is an essential issue for spermatogenesis development. For this reason, piRNAs are considered an important piece in a correct sperm differentiation process. It has been observed in male mice that the interruption of piRNA biosynthesis causes infertility, with non-functional sperm cells. Generally, piRNAs are classified as prepachytene and pachytene piRNAs, depending on the spermatogenesis stage in which they are synthesized (35). Expression of prepachytene piRNAs has been detected in spermatogonia since fetal stages. These piRNAs can be generated either by the *primary* or the *secondary* "ping-pong" mechanisms (32). They are associated with either MIWI2 or MILI proteins (36). It has been observed that the absence of these proteins causes the activation and hypomethylation of transposable elements, such as IAP (Intracisternal A-partile) and LINE1. For this reason, it has been suggested that these PIWI proteins contribute to suppress transposon transcription either by promoting the methylation of their DNA loci, or by eliminating them post-transcriptionally through piRNA action. Additionally, MIWI2 is directly involved in piRNA synthesis from antisense transposable sequences, acting as a counter mechanism for deleting these active retrotransposons (35). Regarding pachytene piRNAs biosynthesis, it can only occur by the *primary* mechanism (32). These piRNAs are attached to MILI or MIWI, which can only act at a post-transcriptional level by silencing transposable elements, without altering methylation patterns (35).

Regulatory role of endo-siRNA during sperm differentiation is not well characterized yet. Nevertheless, it has been suggested that they also take part in spermatogenesis regulation since hundreds of possible targets have been found to be expressed in male germ cells during the whole spermatogenetic process (28).

9.5 SPERM ncRNA INVOLVED IN EMBRYO DEVELOPMENT

Besides providing the paternal genome, human sperm contribution at fertilization also includes additional elements that are essential for early embryo activation and development. They comprise centrioles and proteins from the perinuclear theca of the sperm head, such as phospholipase C-Z (PLC-Z), kinase signaling molecules, transcriptional factors, and structural proteins (37). Among these elements released to the oocyte, sperm RNAs have always been considered a remnant of late spermatogenesis transcription. Therefore, its functionality within the embryo had initially been questioned (38). One of the main reasons for this positioning was the limited amount of sperm RNA that is provided to the zygote (10–20 fg in humans) compared to the total oocyte RNA content (about 330,000 fg in humans) (39,40). Nevertheless, outcomes from multiple studies have proved that sperm RNAs can still be functional in the zygote. In particular, sncRNAs are involved in gene expression regulation during early embryo development.

It has been described that sperm miRNAs and piRNAs remain intact after being released into the oocyte until the start of embryo genome activation (37). Some targets of sperm-specific miRNAs have been detected in metaphase II oocytes in mice (41). Moreover, it has also been observed that miRNAs introduce epigenetic modifications in early embryo stages. An example of these mechanisms would be paramutations: Non-Mendelian mutations produced when the epigenetic alterations of one allele (paramutagenic allele) are transferred to the other one (paramutable allele). This transmission results in modification of gene expression in this paramutable allele. These epigenetic imprints remain even when the paramutagenic allele is gone (42).

9.6 BIOMARKERS OF MALE FERTILITY

Around 15% of couples of reproductive age are affected by infertility. Within this population, male factor is involved in 50% of the cases (43). In spite of the progresses and implementation of new diagnosis techniques during the last decade, there is still a high percentage of men who endure idiopathic infertility of unknown origin (30% of infertile cases) (44). Seminogram analysis constitutes the main approach for male infertility diagnosis, and it is based on observable factors like sperm motility, morphology, or count. The principal handicap of this method is that these measures are not valid indicators in cases of infertile men with normal semen parameters. For this reason, several research lines have been focused on the pursuit of new molecular diagnostic tools. One of the principal fields of interest in this area entails the study of the sperm transcriptome. In this sense, differential and specific expression patterns have been detected in infertile populations. It has been suggested that expression alterations of diverse RNA molecules in infertile patients could be used as biomarkers for diagnostic purposes (45).

Although most of these research studies focus in coding RNAs, an increasing interest in the role of sperm miRNAs has recently emerged based on the marked regulatory nature of these molecules. Comparative analyses between the transcriptome of fertile and infertile patients (asthenozoospermic and oligoasthenozoospermic) was performed by microarray, revealing the overexpression of certain miRNAs (50 in asthenozoospermic and 42 in oligoasthenozoospermic) and the downregulation of others (27 in asthenozoospermic and 44 in asthenozoospermic) (46). Five of these miRNAs (miR-34b*, miR-34b, miR-34c-5p, miR-429, and miR-122) were validated by qRT-PCR and proposed by the authors as a panel of fertility biomarkers (47). Another study compared the sperm miRNA expression levels between fertile and asthenozoospermic patients, and suggested miR-27b as a biomarker of low sperm motility. This miRNA directly regulates the expression of *CRISP2* gene (cysteine-rich secretory protein 2), which is under expressed in asthenozoospermic patients (48). Moreover, Salas-Huetos et al. compared the miRNA profiles between fertile controls and individuals with asthenozoospermia, teratozoospermia, oligozoospermia, and infertile normozoospermia (22,49,50). In these groups of individuals, differential sperm miRNA profiles were associated with the specific fertility problems present in each population. Regarding the biomarker research for other reproductive pathologies, some authors have detected a differential expression of miR-15a in varicocele patients (51).

9.7 CONCLUSIONS

During the last decades, it has been demonstrated that the role of sperm RNAs in male fertility transgresses the preconceived notion that these molecules solely constitute a residual pool from spermatogenesis. Beyond the importance of the protein-coding RNA fraction, discovery of sperm ncRNA functionality revealed a complex regulation net that participates through the whole spermatogenesis process up to early embryonic stages. The intricate pathways of post-transcriptional expression regulation and epigenetic modifications performed by ncRNAs constitute a research topic of special interest. Besides the understanding of the biological relevance of these molecules, many research lines have started to delve into their potential biomarker applications regarding the contribution of the male factor to fertilization and embryo development. Sperm expression studies provide a wide range of opportunities for the establishment of molecular clinical approaches.

REFERENCES

1. Jodar M, Selvaraju S, Sendler E, Diamond MP, Krawetz SA. The presence, role and clinical use of spermatozoal RNAs. *Hum Reprod Update.* 2013;19(6):604–24.
2. Hosken DJ, Hodgson DJ. Why do sperm carry RNA? Relatedness, conflict, and control. *Trends Ecol Evol.* 2014;29(8):451–5.
3. Hamatani T. Human spermatozoal RNAs. *Fertil Steril.* 2012;97(2):275–81.
4. Goodrich R, Anton E, Krawetz S. Isolating mRNA and small noncoding RNAs from human sperm. *Methods Mol Biol.* 2013;927:385–96.
5. Luk ACS, Chan WY, Rennert OM, Lee TL. Long noncoding RNAs in spermatogenesis: Insights from recent high-throughput transcriptome studies. *Reproduction.* 2014;147(5):R131–41.
6. Bao J, Wu J, Schuster AS, Hennig GW, Yan W. Expression profiling reveals developmentally regulated lncRNA repertoire in the mouse male germline. *Biol Reprod.* 2013;89(5):1–12.
7. Kraus P, Sivakamasundari V, Lim SL, Xing X, Lipovich L, Lufkin T. Making sense of Dlx1 antisense RNA. *Dev Biol.* 2013;376(2):224–35.
8. Berghoff EG, Clark MF, Chen S, Cajigas I, Leib DE, Kohtz JD. Evf2 (Dlx6as) lncRNA regulates ultraconserved enhancer methylation and the differential transcriptional control of adjacent genes. *Development.* 2013;140(21):4407–16.
9. Yap KL, Li S, Muñoz-Cabello AM, Raguz S, Zeng L, Gil J et al. Molecular interplay of the non-coding RNA ANRIL and methylated histone H3 lysine 27 by Polycomb CBX7 in transcriptional silencing of INK4a. *Mol Cell.* 2010;38(5):662–74.
10. Klattenhoff CA, Scheuermann JC, Surface LE, Bradley RK, Fields PA, Steinhauser ML et al. Braveheart, a long noncoding RNA required for cardiovascular lineage commitment. *Cell.* 2013;152(3):570–83.

11. Keniry A, Oxley D, Monnier P, Kyba M, Dandolo L, Smits G et al. The H19 lincRNA is a developmental reservoir of miR-675 that suppresses growth and Igf1r. *Nat Cell Biol.* 2012;14(7):659–65.

12. Röther S, Meister G. Small RNAs derived from longer non-coding RNAs. *Biochimie.* 2011;93(11):1905–15.

13. Krawetz SA, Kruger A, Lalancette C, Tagett R, Anton E, Draghici S et al. A survey of small RNAs in human sperm. *Hum Reprod.* 2011;26(12):3401–12.

14. Luo L-F, Hou C-C, Yang W-X. Small non-coding RNAs and their associated proteins in spermatogenesis. *Gene.* 2015;578(2):141–57.

15. Place R, Li L, Pookot D, Noonan E, Dahiya R. MicroRNA-373 induces expression of genes with complementary promoter sequences. *Proc Natl Acad Sci USA.* 2008;105:1608–13.

16. Cai X, Hagedorn CH, Cullen BR. Human microRNAs are processed from capped, polyadenylated transcripts that can also function as mRNAs. *RNA.* 2004;10:1957–66.

17. Ambros V. microRNAs: Tiny regulators with great potential. *Cell.* 2001;107:823–6.

18. Schwarz DS, Hutvágner G, Du T, Xu Z, Aronin N, Zamore PD. Asymmetry in the assembly of the RNAi enzyme complex. *Cell.* 2003;115(2):199–208.

19. Ro S, Park C, Sanders KMK, McCarrey JR, Yan W, McCarrey J et al. Cloning and expression profiling of testis-expressed microRNAs. *Dev Biol.* 2007;311(2):592–602.

20. Thomas M, Lieberman J, Lal A. Desperately seeking microRNA targets. *Nat Struct Mol Biol.* 2010;17(10):1169–74.

21. Luo L, Ye L, Liu G, Shao G, Zheng R, Ren Z et al. Microarray-Based approach identifies differentially expressed MicroRNAs in porcine sexually immature and mature testes. *PLoS One.* 2010;5(8):e11744.

22. Salas-Huetos A, Blanco J, Vidal F, Mercader JM, Garrido N, Anton E. New insights into the expression profile and function of micro-ribonucleic acid in human spermatozoa. *Fertil Steril.* 2014;102(1):213–22.

23. Ostermeier GC, Goodrich RJ, Diamond MP, Dix DJ, Krawetz SA. Toward using stable spermatozoal RNAs for prognostic assessment of male factor fertility. *Fertil Steril.* 2005;83(6):1687–94.

24. Chuma S, Nakano T. piRNA and spermatogenesis in mice. *Philos Trans R Soc Lond B Biol Sci.* 2013;368(1609):20110338.

25. Pantano L, Jodar M, Bak M, Ballescà JL, Tommerup N, Oliva R et al. The small RNA content of human sperm reveals pseudogene-derived piRNAs complementary to protein-coding genes. *RNA.* 2015;21(6):1085–95.

26. Girard A, Sachidanandam R, Hannon GJ, Carmell MA. A germline-specific class of small RNAs binds mammalian Piwi proteins. *Nature.* 2006;442(7099):199–202.

27. Song R, Hennig GW, Wu Q, Jose C, Zheng H, Yan W. Male germ cells express abundant endogenous siRNAs. *Proc Natl Acad Sci USA.* 2011;108(32):13159–64.

28. Suh N, Baehner L, Moltzahn F, Melton C, Chen J, Blelloch R. MicroRNA function is globally suppressed in mouse oocytes and early embryos. *Curr Biol.* 2010;20(3):271–7.

29. Dadoune J. Spermatozoal RNAs: What about their functions? *Microsc Res Tech.* 2009;72(8):536–51.

30. Cappallo-Obermann H, Schulze W, Jastrow H, Baukloh V, Spiess A. Highly purified spermatozoal RNA obtained by a novel method indicates an un- usual 28S/18S rRNA ratio and suggests impaired ribosome assembly. *Mol Hum Reprod.* 2011;17(11):669–78.

31. Miller D, Ostermeier GC, Krawetz SA. The controversy, potential and roles of spermatozoal RNA. *Trends Mol Med.* 2005;11(4):156–63.

32. De Mateo S, Sassone-corsi P. Regulation of spermatogenesis by small non-coding RNAs: Role of the germ granule. *Semin Cell Dev Biol.* 2014;29:84–92.

33. Kotaja N. MicroRNAs and spermatogenesis. *Fertil Steril.* 2014;101(6):1552–62.

34. Tong M-H, Mitchell D, Evanoff R, Griswold MD. Expression of mirlet7 family microRNAs in response to retinoic acid-induced spermatogonial differentiation in mice. *Biol Reprod.* 2011;85(1):189–97.

35. Pillai RS, Chuma S. piRNAs and their involvement in male germline development in mice. *Dev Growth Differ.* 2012;54:78–92.

36. Yadav RP, Kotaja N. Small RNAs in spermatogenesis. *Mol Cell Endocrinol.* 2014;382(1):498–508.

37. Boerke A, Dieleman S, Gadella B. A possible role for sperm RNA in early embryo development. *Theriogenology.* 2007;68S:147–55.

38. Cummins J. Cytoplasmic inheritance and its implications for animal biotechnology. *Theriogenology.* 2001;55(6):1381–99.

39. Kocabas AM, Crosby J, Ross PJ, Otu HH, Beyhan Z, Can H et al. The transcriptome of human oocytes. *Proc Natl Acad Sci USA.* 2006;103(38):14027–32.

40. Krawetz S. Paternal contribution: New insights and future challenges. *Nat Rev Genet.* 2005;6(8):633–42.

41. Amanai M, Brahmajosyula M, Perry A. A restricted role for sperm-borne microRNAs in mammalian fertilization. *Biol Reprod.* 2006;75(6):877–84.

42. Pilu R. Paramutation: Just a curiosity or fine tuning of gene expression in the next generation? *Curr Genomics.* 2011;12:298–306.

43. Dohle G, Colpi G, Hargreave T, Papp G, Jungwirth A, Weidner W. EAU guidelines on male infertility. *Eur Urol.* 2005;48(5):703–11.

44. Ray A, Shah A, Gudi A, Homburg R. Unexplained infertility: An update and review of practice. *Reprod Biomed Online.* 2012;24(6):591–602.

45. Anton E, Krawetz S. Spermatozoa as biomarkers for the assessment of human male infertility and genotoxicity. *Syst Biol Reprod Med.* 2012;58(1):41–50.

46. Abu-Halima M, Hammadeh M, Schmitt J, Leidinger P, Keller A, Meese E et al. Altered microRNA expression profiles of human spermatozoa in patients with different spermatogenic impairments. *Fertil Steril.* 2013;99(5):1249–55.

47. Abu-Halima M, Hammadeh M, Backes C, Fischer U, Leidinger P, Lubbad AM et al. Panel of five microRNAs as potential biomarkers for the diagnosis and assessment of male infertility. *Fertil Steril.* 2014;102(4):989–97.

48. Zhou J-H, Zhou QZ, Lyu X-M, Zhu T, Chen Z-J, Chen M-K et al. The expression of cysteine-rich secretory protein 2 (CRISP2) and its specific regulator miR-27b in the spermatozoa of patients with asthenozoospermia. *Biol Reprod.* 2015;92(1):1–9.

49. Salas-Huetos A, Blanco J, Vidal F, Godo A, Grossmann M, Pons MC et al. Spermatozoa from patients with seminal alterations exhibit a differential micro-ribonucleic acid profile. *Fertil Steril.* 2015;104(3):591–601.

50. Salas-Huetos A, Blanco J, Vidal F, Grossmann M, Pons MC, Garrido N et al. Sperm from normozoospermic fertile and infertile individuals convey a distinct miRNA cargo. *Andrology.* 2016;4:1028–36.

51. Ji Z, Lu R, Mou L, Duan YG, Zhang Q, Wang Y et al. Expressions of miR-15a and its target gene HSPA1B in the spermatozoa of patients with varicocele. *Reproduction.* 2014;147(5):693–701.

Epigenetic and Assisted Reproduction Experimental Studies

Ovarian Stimulation

Patricia Fauque

CONTENTS

10.1 INTRODUCTION

Almost 10% of couples are infertile (1) and providing them with safe techniques to reach parenthood is a public health issue. The two most common types of assisted reproductive technologies (ART) are conventional *in vitro* fertilization (IVF) and intracytoplasmic sperm injection (ICSI), which are accompanied by three major procedures: (1) controlled ovarian hyperstimulation, (2) *in vitro* fertilization, and (3) embryo culture (Figure 10.1). They account for >1% of births in the United States (2), and >4% of births in some European countries (3). Although these techniques are thought to be generally safe, evidence suggests they carry an increased risk of adverse perinatal outcomes and morbid congenital problems (4). Furthermore, although findings are contradictory (5–9), several reports have pointed

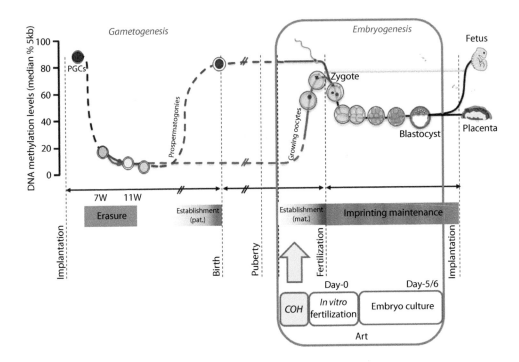

FIGURE 10.1 Reproductive procedures (ART) involving three major procedures (i.e., controlled ovarian hyperstimulation, *in vitro* fertilization, and embryo culture) coincide with DNA methylation changes taking place during gametogenesis and embryogenesis. The progenitors of the human germline (PGCs, primordial germ cells) undergo a marked first genome-wide DNA demethylation (levels are less than 10%) (56). After the period of demethylation, male germ cells initiate and complete the remethylation during prenatal development until puberty (57–59). In contrast, oocytes in the female, arrested at the prophase of meiosis I, remain hypomethylated throughout the fetal period (57–59). After puberty, DNA methylation is then acquired during the growing phase of the oocyte cohort from the primary to the antral follicle stage (23). Controlled ovarian hyperstimulation (COH) thus leads to the development of multiple oocytes and occurs simultaneously with the reprogramming of the oocyte genome. Following fertilization, maternal and paternal epigenomes introduced by the gametes must be reset a second time (second wave) to establish the pluripotency that is required for the development of embryonic lineages (60). In contrast, the imprinting control regions (ICRs) of imprinted genes escape demethylation (61). Parental-specific DNA methylation of ICRs is acquired in the germline (Establishment phase) and must remain after fertilization (Imprinting maintenance phase).

toward an increased risk of diseases caused by abnormal genomic imprinting such as Beckwith-Wiedemann (BWS), Russell-Silver (RS), and Angelman (AS) syndromes (10–12).

This excess of developmental anomalies and imprinting disorders following ART, as well as the fact that all ART-BWS cases typically occur though loss of DNA methylation in imprinting control regions (ICRs) suggests that ART techniques are associated with potential epigenetic risks, although the infertility/subfertility status of the parents may also play a role in the increased incidence of these disorders (13). Indeed, ART procedures take place when major epigenetic reprogramming is occurring, especially during female gametogenesis and after fertilization (Figure 10.1).

Reprogramming of the epigenome, which involves dynamic DNA methylation changes in particular, is essential for the acquisition and maintenance of gametic identity, pluripotency, and embryonic lineage decisions, but one other major outcome of this is genomic imprinting. Genomic imprinting is an epigenetic process, whereby a subset of genes, called "imprinted genes" (IGs) are preferentially expressed by one parental chromosome. Notably, genomic imprinting is characterized by the acquisition of sex-specific marks (DNA methylation being the most often described) on regulatory sequences referred to as imprinting control regions (ICRs) in the germline (*Establishment phase*). These marks must remain after fertilization (*Imprinting maintenance phase*) (Figure 10.1). In female gametogenesis, these marks, which are catalyzed by the DNA methyltransferase family of enzymes (DNMTs), are acquired during the oocyte growth phase. After fertilization, these ICRs act in *cis* to achieve complete or partial monoallelic expression of most IGs. Although IGs account for a very small number of genes (approximately 150 imprinted genes have been identified in mice and humans (14–16) (http://www.geneimprint.com/site/genes-by-species), they exert crucial roles in embryonic/fetal growth and development, including placentation (17), postnatal metabolic pathways and behavior associated with the control of resources (18).

As developed in this review, one important procedure with regard to possible epigenetic alterations is ovarian stimulation. First, the observation of epigenetic disorders in children conceived after the IVF and ICSI techniques as well as IUI, with/or without donor sperm, supports this notion (19). In addition, in some patients with BWS or AS, the only ART procedure used was ovarian stimulation (20–22). Second, in oogenesis, DNA methylation at ICRs begins after puberty in growing oocytes, from primordial to antral follicles when ovarian stimulation is administered. The use of exogenous hormones during this period may disrupt the acquisition of imprints in oocyte maturation. Interestingly, most of the ICRs are methylated in the oocyte (19 maternal ICRs from 23 currently identified) whereas only four have been found in sperm (paternal ICRs) (14–16). Due to this high number of maternal ICRs, the frequency of imprinting errors during maternal epigenetic reprogramming is statistically higher than that in sperm. Moreover, in order to produce an increased number of ovulated oocytes in IVF or ICSI treatments, the doses of hormones delivered to achieve ovarian stimulation are higher than those found in spontaneous ovulation or even with IUI treatments notably, especially in cases of female infertility with low ovarian reserve or in advanced maternal age. This forced oocyte maturation may lead to the loss of maternal-specific expression and the development of imprinting disorders in some oocytes that in normal conditions would not be ovulated (23). Third, experimental animal studies detailed in this review have demonstrated that ovarian stimulation can disrupt the mechanism that maintains DNA methylation of ICRs in the preimplantation embryo.

10.2 EPIGENETIC EFFECTS OF OVARIAN STIMULATION: EXPERIMENTAL MOUSE STUDIES

Experimental studies in mice have demonstrated that ART procedures can perturb embryonic development and lead to increased embryo loss, reduced litter size, and decreased fetal weight (24). It is therefore hypothesized that ART procedures could disrupt the mechanism that maintains DNA methylation of ICRs in the preimplantation embryo. In support of this argument, we and others have investigated procedures used in ART using a mouse model and have linked some reproductive procedures to loss of DNA methylation at ICRs and/or aberrant expression of IGs at the blastocyst stage or later in extraembryonic tissues (23–34).

Concerning the superovulation effects per se, epigenetic modifications on IGs were mainly not observed in the gametes but later at the blastocyst stage or during the gestation (Table 10.1). Indeed, overall, we found expected imprinted methylation patterns of several IGs (*maternal* IGs for which the percentage of DNA methylation is close to 100% such as *Snrpn*, *Peg3*, and *Kcnq1ot1*; *paternal* IGs for which the percentage of DNA methylation is close to 0% such as *H19*) in individual or pooled mature oocytes from superovulated female mice (35,36). However, these results may vary as superovulated mature oocytes show heterogeneous DNA methylation of maternal IGs, suggesting that the methylation imprint may not be established in all oocytes obtained after superovulation (50).

By contrast, the effects of superovulation on epigenetics have been observed in embryos before implantation. As an example, one report showed that ovarian stimulation can alter

TABLE 10.1   Effects of Superovulation on Imprinted Gene Expression and Methylation in Mouse Preimplanted Embryos

Control Group	Manipulation Groups	Gene	Results of Expression Analysis	Results of Methylation Analysis	Ref.
In vivo	SO (blastocysts)	*H19*	↓	No LOM	(25)
In vivo	SO (low and high hormone dosages) (blastocysts)	*Snrpn*	NA	Maternal allele LOM, dose-dependent	(62)
		Peg3	NA	Maternal allele LOM, dose-dependent	
		Kcnq1ot1	NA	Maternal allele LOM, dose-dependent	
		H19	NA	Maternal allele GOM, dose-dependent Paternal allele LOM, dose-dependent	
In vivo	SO (16-cell embryos)	*H19* and *Snrpn*	NA	No LOM	(27)

Abbreviations: GOM = Gain of methylation; LOM = loss of methylation; NA = not analyzed; SO = super-ovulation; ↓ = decreased compared with control.

H19 DNA methylation (i.e., hypomethylation of the *H19* paternal allele), leading to its misexpression in mouse blastocysts (25,26). Interestingly, these imprinting errors occurred in a dose-dependent manner, with more frequent disturbances after high than after low hormone doses. Accordingly, abnormal global DNA methylation patterns, assessed by either methylcytosine immunofluorescence or repeat-element analysis, were observed in embryos from superovulated as compared to those from non-superovulated females (37,38).

Several teams also found these epigenetic alterations after implantation of the embryo, mainly in placental tissue (29,34,39) (Table 10.2). Keeping the *H19* gene example, placentas displayed active expression of the normally silent *H19* allele.

Finally, this indicates that impairment of imprinting mechanisms resulting from superovulation (herein, the molecular machinery involved in the maintenance of DNA methylation) can persist in later stages of intrauterine development and could have a direct

TABLE 10.2   Effects of Superovulation on Feto-Placental Development and on Imprinted Gene Expression and Methylation in Concepti and/or Placentas of Mice

GA Study	Control Group	Manipulation Group	Weight		Results of Expression Analysis		Results of Methylation Analysis		Ref.
			F	P	F	P	F	P	
E9.5	*In vivo* fertilization	SO, blastocyst transfer	NA	NA	Monoallelic: H19, Cdkn1c, Kcnq1, Ascl2, Zim1, Snrpn, Kcnq1ot1, Peg3, Igf2, Mkrn3	Biallelic: *H19* High levels of misexpression: at least 1/8 IG ↑ Ascl2, = H19 ↓ Igf2	NA	NA	(34)
E9.5	*In vivo* fertilization	SO	NA	NA	Monoallelic: H19, Snrpn, Igf2, Kncq1ot1 = Igf2	Biallelic: H19, Snrpn Monoallelic: Igf2, Kncq1ot1 ↑ Igf2	NA	= H19, Snrpn	(29)
	Blastocyst transfer	SO, blastocyst transfer	NA	NA	Monoallelic: H19, Snrpn, Igf2 = Igf2	Biallelic: H19 Monoallelic: Snrpn, Igf2 ↑ Igf2	NA	= H19, Snrpn	
E18.5	*In vivo* fertilization	SO, blastocyst transfer	=	↑		↓ Glut3 =Glut1, Snat2, Snat4, Snrpn, Peg3, Kcnq1ot1	NA	=Snat4, Glut3, H19, Peg3	(63)

Abbreviations: E = Embryonic day; F = Fetus; GA = Gestational Age; NA = Not Analyzed; P = Placenta; SO = SuperOvulation; ↑ = increased; ↓ = decreased; "=" = no significant difference compared with control.

effect on intrauterine growth as observed in ART-offspring. Notably, perturbations of DNA methylation following superovulation and embryo transfer have been observed in mice, particularly in the placenta, and resulted in birth defects in the offspring (39).

However, these stochastic epimutations are corrected in the germline of adult male mice produced using superovulation and are not reproduced in their progenies (40). These results in mice (in line with our findings in humans [41]) indicate that germline-related epigenetic reprogramming limits in general the transmission of primary methylation errors to subsequent generations.

10.3 EPIGENETIC EFFECTS OF OVARIAN STIMULATION: HUMAN STUDIES

Due to ethical reasons, few studies have been conducted in humans, especially on mature oocytes. In addition, important confounders such as the woman's age and subfertility make research in this field more complex, and explain discrepant results in the literature. Even though some authors found normal methylation profiles for a maternal IG (i.e., *SNRPN* gene -(42), others reported imprinted errors for *PEG1* (loss of methylation) and *H19* (gain of methylation) genes but without being able to determine whether they were due to the ovarian stimulation, maternal age or oocyte maturation stage or if they were inherent to female subfertility (43).

However, the results from the only human study to analyze oocytes from natural and stimulated cycles (44) suggest that gonadotropin stimulation may modify the dynamics of *de novo* methylation during oocyte maturation and/or may recruit follicles that are too young (23). These imprint disruptions may be caused by the delayed/accelerated development of oocytes, thus preventing/perturbing the establishment of imprints in oocytes at the right time.

To date, the one study which had the unique opportunity to separate the possible effects of ovarian stimulation did not report any differences in methylation at imprinted loci in placenta or cord blood of infants conceived with ovarian stimulation compared with infants conceived spontaneously (9).

10.4 EPIGENETIC EFFECTS OF OVARIAN STIMULATION ON THE ENDOMETRIUM

Evidence from superovulated mice shows that hormonal stimulation is associated with a high risk of fetal growth retardation and an increased number of embryonic resorptions (29,45,46). Apart from the effects of ovarian stimulation on gametes and embryos, this procedure may induce epigenetic modifications in the endometrium. It is well known that hormonal treatments in humans modify the maturation of the endometrium (47,48) as well as the global expression profiles in the endometrium in a dose-dependent manner (49,50). Thus, as DNA methylation is involved in endometrial receptivity and decidualization (51,52), hormonal treatments could modify these processes. Interestingly, different expression patterns of DNA methytransferases (DNMT1, 3a,3b) were observed and were dependent on the period of the reproductive cycle in both humans (53,54) and mice (55).

These findings provide support for the potential role of DNA methylation in endometrial changes during embryo implantation after hormonal treatments. Further experiments are needed to clarify the impact of ovarian stimulation on endometrial DNA methylation and implantation failure processes.

10.5 CONCLUSION

To date, it is unclear which ART procedures are involved in epigenetic anomalies. However, the fact that epigenetic disorders occur in children conceived using IVF/IUI techniques, even when the only ART procedure used was ovarian stimulation (20–22), supports the notion that ovarian stimulation could be involved. Another argument in favor of hormonal epigenetic disruption is that the DNA methylation marks are laid down at different times in male and female gametogenesis. DNA methylation acquisition at DMRs occurs during prenatal stages of spermatogenesis and is completed at the postnatal stage, whereas in oogenesis it begins later after puberty in growing oocytes, from primordial to antral follicles. Ovarian stimulation using exogeneous hormones administered during this period may disrupt the acquisition of imprints in oocyte maturation. Moreover, in order to produce an increased number of ovulated oocytes in IVF or ICSI treatments, the dose of hormones to achieve ovarian stimulation are higher than those found in spontaneous ovulation or when IUI treatments are used. This forced oocyte maturation may lead to the loss of maternal-specific expression and the development of imprinting disorders in some oocytes that in normal conditions would not be ovulated. It is extremely difficult in humans to distinguish between the effects of ovarian stimulation and those of other infertility-contributing factors on genomic imprinting. However, mouse studies highlighted the deleterious effects on epigenetics (specifically, on genomic imprinting). Thus, deleterious effects of hormonal treatments may alter epigenetic reprogramming during the maturation of oocytes. However, as developed in this review, induced ovarian stimulation may also modify the physiological environment of the uterus and the implantation. Moreover, ART techniques could also exacerbate detrimental developmental and epigenetic outcomes in a context of compromised oocyte quality. Such a phenomenon was recently demonstrated in the mouse model (39). Other epigenetic mechanisms may also be affected by ovarian stimulation, such as histone modifications, which are known to play an important role in placental epigenetic regulation. Therefore, the research focus should shift toward these processes.

All in all, these results should encourage researchers to analyze the effects of potential epigenetic changes of gametes/endometrium related to ovarian stimulation on the epigenetic setting of the conceptus in humans, and strive to minimize these variations in the interest of epigenetic safety after ART. Notably, as in humans it is not possible to avoid the cumulative effects of ART procedures, an effort should be made to decrease doses of exogeneous hormones as much as possible.

REFERENCES

1. Boivin J, Bunting L, Collins JA, Nygren KG. International estimates of infertility prevalence and treatment-seeking: Potential need and demand for infertility medical care. *Hum Reprod.* 2007;22(6):1506–12.
2. Dyer S, Chambers GM, de Mouzon J et al. International committee for monitoring assisted reproductive technologies world report. Assisted reproductive technology 2008, 2009, and 2010. *Hum Reprod.* 2016;31(7):1588–609.
3. European IVFMCftESoHR, Embryology, Calhaz-Jorge C et al. Assisted reproductive technology in Europe, 2012: Results generated from European registers by ESHRE. *Hum Reprod.* 2016;31(8):1638–52.
4. Ceelen M, van Weissenbruch MM, Vermeiden JP et al. Growth and development of children born after *in vitro* fertilization. *Fertil Steril.* 2008;90(5):1662–73.
5. Bowdin S, Allen C, Kirby G et al. A survey of assisted reproductive technology births and imprinting disorders. *Hum Reprod.* 2007;22(12):3237–40.
6. Kallen B, Finnstrom O, Nygren KG, Olausson PO. *In vitro* fertilization (IVF) in Sweden: Infant outcome after different IVF fertilization methods. *Fertil Steril.* 2005;84(3):611–7.
7. Manning M, Lissens W, Bonduelle M et al. Study of DNA-methylation patterns at chromosome 15q11-q13 in children born after ICSI reveals no imprinting defects. *Mol Hum Reprod.* 2000;6(11):1049–53.
8. Tierling S, Souren NY, Gries J et al. Assisted reproductive technologies do not enhance the variability of DNA methylation imprints in human. *J Med Genet.* 2010;47(6):371–6.
9. Rancourt RC, Harris HR, Michels KB. Methylation levels at imprinting control regions are not altered with ovulation induction or *in vitro* fertilization in a birth cohort. *Hum Reprod.* 2012;27(7):2208–16.
10. Jammes H, Fauque P, Jouannet P. [Contribution of animal models to the study of reproduction, assisted reproductive technologies and of development]. *Bull Acad Natl Med.* 2010;194(2):301–17; discussion 17–8.
11. Lazaraviciute G, Kauser M, Bhattacharya S, Haggarty P. A systematic review and meta-analysis of DNA methylation levels and imprinting disorders in children conceived by IVF/ICSI compared with children conceived spontaneously. *Hum Reprod Update.* 2014;20(6):840–52.
12. Vermeiden JP, Bernardus RE. Are imprinting disorders more prevalent after human *in vitro* fertilization or intracytoplasmic sperm injection? *Fertil Steril.* 2013;99(3):642–51.
13. Doornbos ME, Maas SM, McDonnell J et al. Infertility, assisted reproduction technologies and imprinting disturbances: A Dutch study. *Hum Reprod.* 2007;22(9):2476–80.
14. Barbaux S, Gascoin-Lachambre G, Buffat C et al. A genome-wide approach reveals novel imprinted genes expressed in the human placenta. *Epigenetics.* 2012;7(9):1079–90.
15. Proudhon C, Duffie R, Ajjan S et al. Protection against de novo methylation is instrumental in maintaining parent-of-origin methylation inherited from the gametes. *Mol Cell.* 2012;47(6):909–20.

16. Court F, Tayama C, Romanelli V et al. Genome-wide parent-of-origin DNA methylation analysis reveals the intricacies of human imprinting and suggests a germline methylation-independent mechanism of establishment. *Genome Res.* 2014;24(4):554–69.

17. Tunster SJ, Jensen AB, John RM. Imprinted genes in mouse placental development and the regulation of fetal energy stores. *Reproduction.* 2013;145(5):R117–37.

18. Constancia M, Kelsey G, Reik W. Resourceful imprinting. *Nature.* 2004;432(7013):53–7.

19. Montfoort APAv. Epigenetics and assisted reproductive technology. *Textbook of human reproductive genetics* 2014. doi:10.1017/CBO9781139236027.013.

20. Sutcliffe AG, Peters CJ, Bowdin S et al. Assisted reproductive therapies and imprinting disorders—A preliminary British survey. *Hum Reprod.* 2006;21(4):1009–11.

21. Ludwig H. Archives of gynecology and obstetrics: 135 years. *Arch Gynecol Obstet.* 2005;271(1):1–5.

22. Chang AS, Moley KH, Wangler M, Feinberg AP, Debaun MR. Association between Beckwith-Wiedemann syndrome and assisted reproductive technology: A case series of 19 patients. *Fertility and sterility.* 2005;83(2):349–54.

23. Fauque P. Ovulation induction and epigenetic anomalies. *Fertil Steril.* 2013;99(3):616–23.

24. Choux C, Carmignac V, Bruno C et al. The placenta: Phenotypic and epigenetic modifications induced by assisted reproductive technologies throughout pregnancy. *Clin Epigenetics.* 2015;7:87.

25. Fauque P, Jouannet P, Lesaffre C et al. Assisted reproductive technology affects developmental kinetics, H19 imprinting control region methylation and H19 gene expression in individual mouse embryos. *BMC Dev Biol.* 2007;7:116.

26. Market-Velker BA, Fernandes AD, Mann MR. Side-by-side comparison of five commercial media systems in a mouse model: Suboptimal *in vitro* culture interferes with imprint maintenance. *Biol Reprod.* 2010;83(6):938–50.

27. El Hajj N, Trapphoff T, Linke M et al. Limiting dilution bisulphite (pyro)sequencing reveals parent-specific methylation patterns in single early mouse embryos and bovine oocytes. *Epigenetics.* 2011;6(10):1176–88.

28. de Waal E, Yamazaki Y, Ingale P et al. Gonadotropin stimulation contributes to an increased incidence of epimutations in ICSI-derived mice. *Hum Mol Genet.* 2012;21(20):4460–72.

29. Fortier AL, Lopes FL, Darricarrere N et al. Superovulation alters the expression of imprinted genes in the midgestation mouse placenta. *Hum Mol Genet.* 2008;17(11):1653–65.

30. de Waal E, Mak W, Calhoun S et al. *In vitro* culture increases the frequency of stochastic epigenetic errors at imprinted genes in placental tissues from mouse concepti produced through assisted reproductive technologies. *Biol Reprod.* 2014;90(2):22.

31. Fauque P, Mondon F, Letourneur F et al. *In vitro* fertilization and embryo culture strongly impact the placental transcriptome in the mouse model. *PLoS One.* 2010;5(2):e9218.

32. Fauque P, Ripoche MA, Tost J et al. Modulation of imprinted gene network in placenta results in normal development of *in vitro* manipulated mouse embryos. *Hum Mol Genet.* 2010;19(9):1779–90.

33. Mann MR, Lee SS, Doherty AS et al. Selective loss of imprinting in the placenta following preimplantation development in culture. *Development.* 2004;131(15):3727–35.

34. Rivera RM, Stein P, Weaver JR et al. Manipulations of mouse embryos prior to implantation result in aberrant expression of imprinted genes on day 9.5 of development. *Hum Mol Genet.* 2008;17(1):1–14.

35. Anckaert E, Adriaenssens T, Romero S et al. Unaltered imprinting establishment of key imprinted genes in mouse oocytes after *in vitro* follicle culture under variable follicle-stimulating hormone exposure. *Int J Dev Biol.* 2009;53(4):541–8.

36. Denomme MM, Zhang L, Mann MR. Embryonic imprinting perturbations do not originate from superovulation-induced defects in DNA methylation acquisition. *Fertil Steril.* 2011;96(3):734–8 e2.

37. Liang XW, Cui XS, Sun SC et al. Superovulation induces defective methylation in line-1 retrotransposon elements in blastocyst. *Reprod Biol Endocrinol.* 2013;11:69.

38. Shi W, Haaf T. Aberrant methylation patterns at the two-cell stage as an indicator of early developmental failure. *Mol Reprod Dev.* 2002;63(3):329–34.

39. Whidden L, Martel J, Rahimi S et al. Compromised oocyte quality and assisted reproduction contribute to sex-specific effects on offspring outcomes and epigenetic patterning. *Hum Mol Genet.* 2016;25(21):4649–60.

40. de Waal E, Yamazaki Y, Ingale P et al. Primary epimutations introduced during intracytoplasmic sperm injection (ICSI) are corrected by germline-specific epigenetic reprogramming. *Proc Natl Acad Sci USA.* 2012;109(11):4163–8.

41. Bruno C, Carmignac V, Netchine I et al. Germline correction of an epimutation related to Silver-Russell syndrome. *Hum Mol Genet.* 2015;24(12):3314–21.

42. Geuns E, Hilven P, Van Steirteghem A et al. Methylation analysis of KvDMR1 in human oocytes. *J Med Genet.* 2007;44(2):144–7.

43. Sato C, Shimada M, Mori T et al. Assessment of human oocyte developmental competence by cumulus cell morphology and circulating hormone profile. *Reproductive Biomedicine Online.* 2007;14(1):49–56.

44. Khoueiry R, Ibala-Rhomdane S, Mery L et al. Dynamic CpG methylation of the KCNQ1OT1 gene during maturation of human oocytes. *J Med Genet.* 2008;45(9):583–8.

45. Ertzeid G, Storeng R. The impact of ovarian stimulation on implantation and fetal development in mice. *Hum Reprod.* 2001;16(2):221–5.

46. Van der Auwera I, D'Hooghe T. Superovulation of female mice delays embryonic and fetal development. *Hum Reprod.* 2001;16(6):1237–43.

47. Kolibianakis E, Bourgain C, Albano C et al. Effect of ovarian stimulation with recombinant follicle-stimulating hormone, gonadotropin releasing hormone antagonists, and human chorionic gonadotropin on endometrial maturation on the day of oocyte pick-up. *Fertil Steril.* 2002;78(5):1025–9.

48. Nikas G, Develioglu OH, Toner JP, Jones HW Jr. Endometrial pinopodes indicate a shift in the window of receptivity in IVF cycles. *Hum Reprod.* 1999;14(3):787–92.

49. Haouzi D, Assou S, Dechanet C et al. Controlled ovarian hyperstimulation for *in vitro* fertilization alters endometrial receptivity in humans: Protocol effects. *Biol Reprod.* 2010;82(4):679–86.

50. Horcajadas JA, Riesewijk A, Polman J et al. Effect of controlled ovarian hyperstimulation in IVF on endometrial gene expression profiles. *Mol Hum Reprod.* 2005;11(3):195–205.

51. Logan PC, Ponnampalam AP, Rahnama F et al. The effect of DNA methylation inhibitor 5-Aza-2′-deoxycytidine on human endometrial stromal cells. *Hum Reprod.* 2010;25(11):2859–69.

52. Rahnama F, Thompson B, Steiner M et al. Epigenetic regulation of E-cadherin controls endometrial receptivity. *Endocrinology.* 2009;150(3):1466–72.

53. Vincent ZL, Farquhar CM, Mitchell MD, Ponnampalam AP. Expression and regulation of DNA methyltransferases in human endometrium. *Fertil Steril.* 2011;95(4):1522–5 e1.

54. Yamagata Y, Maekawa R, Asada H et al. Aberrant DNA methylation status in human uterine leiomyoma. *Mol Hum Reprod.* 2009;15(4):259–67.

55. Ding YB, He JL, Liu XQ et al. Expression of DNA methyltransferases in the mouse uterus during early pregnancy and susceptibility to dietary folate deficiency. *Reproduction.* 2012;144(1):91–100.

56. von Meyenn F, Reik W. Forget the parents: Epigenetic reprogramming in human germ cells. *Cell.* 2015;161(6):1248–51.

57. Cantone I, Fisher AG. Epigenetic programming and reprogramming during development. *Nat Struct Mol Biol.* 2013;20(3):282–9.

58. Saitou M, Kagiwada S, Kurimoto K. Epigenetic reprogramming in mouse pre-implantation development and primordial germ cells. *Development.* 2012;139(1):15–31.

59. Smallwood SA, Kelsey G. De novo DNA methylation: A germ cell perspective. *Trends Genet.* 2012;28(1):33–42.

60. Reik W, Surani MA. Germline and Pluripotent Stem Cells. *Cold Spring Harb Perspect Biol.* 2015;7(11). pii: a019422.

61. Barlow DP, Bartolomei MS. Genomic imprinting in mammals. *Cold Spring Harb Perspect Biol.* 2014;6(2). pii: a018382.

62. Market-Velker BA, Zhang L, Magri LS et al. Dual effects of superovulation: Loss of maternal and paternal imprinted methylation in a dose-dependent manner. *Hum Mol Genet.* 2010;19(1):36–51.

63. de Waal E, Vrooman LA, Fischer E et al. The cumulative effect of assisted reproduction procedures on placental development and epigenetic perturbations in a mouse model. *Hum Mol Genet.* 2015;24(24):6975–85.

Epigenetic and Assisted Reproduction Experimental Studies

In Vitro Culture

Serafín Pérez-Cerezales, Noelia Fonseca Balvís,

Benjamín Planells, Isabel Gómez-Redondo, Eric

Marqués-García, Ricardo Laguna-Barraza, Eva Pericuesta,

Raul Fernández-González, and Alfonso Gutiérrez-Adán

CONTENTS

11.1 INTRODUCTION

A number of factors can determine the quality, viability, and health of preimplantation embryos produced by assisted reproduction technology (ART). Some of these factors are external and out of the control of the laboratory conducting ART, like the genetics of the patients, their habits such as diet and drug consumption as well as the etiology of each infertility case or the sensitivity to respond to ovarian stimulation, and so on. On the other hand, the ART laboratory can control other variables that are susceptible of improvement such as the composition of the media, the use of protein supplements, the atmosphere of the culture conditions, the density of embryo, the plastic ware used and the use of oil overlay. Thus, for example, the development of culture media for successfully produce preimplantation embryos has had a profound effect improving ART outcome. However, despite all the improvement achieved, preimplantation embryos are still difficult to culture successfully *in vitro*, and this is in part because we still do not know the underlying metabolic changes occurring during early development. Only understanding this process, could we optimize culture media and conditions. Since the introduction of commercially available culture media, there has been a rapid development of different formulations, often with unknown composition due to industrial protection. As consequence of this lack of knowledge and failure in developing optimal culture media, there are many evidences showing that *in vitro* embryo culture (IVC) can produce reprograming of embryonic growth leading to epigenetic alterations in embryos and placenta, producing alterations in fetal growth trajectory, birthweight, childhood growth and long-term disease including Type II diabetes, cardiovascular problems, and so on (1,2) (Figure 11.1). Consequently, it

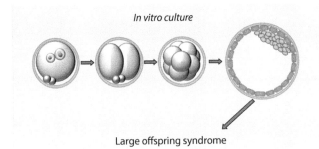

In vitro culture

Large offspring syndrome

- Increased prenatal loss
- Large placentas
- Large fetuses
- Polyhydramnios
- Parturition problems

- Higher perinatal mortality
- Breathing difficulties
- Reluctance to suckle
- Skeletal anomalies
- Large organs
- Cerebellar dysplasia

FIGURE 11.1   IVC of preimplantation embryos has been associated with several disorders in the mouse, human, and cow; as *large offspring syndrome* in the cow that includes excessive birthweight, incorrect placentation, congenital deformities, or even abortion. This syndrome has been related with alteration in methylation of imprinting genes. This association has been observed in several species including loss of imprinting DNA methylation in mouse blastocysts produced by IVC, and in humans, where ART and IVC have been associated with imprinting syndromes, such as Beckwith-Wiedemann, Prader-Willi, and Angelman.

has been reported that IVC also has deleterious long-term effects in mice (3,4) and cows (5) (Figure 11.1).

Unlike differentiated somatic cells, whose epigenetic patterns seem to be stable, epigenetic marks during preimplantation embryos are changing dynamically to maintain cell reprograming during development. Paternal genome undergoes active genome-wide

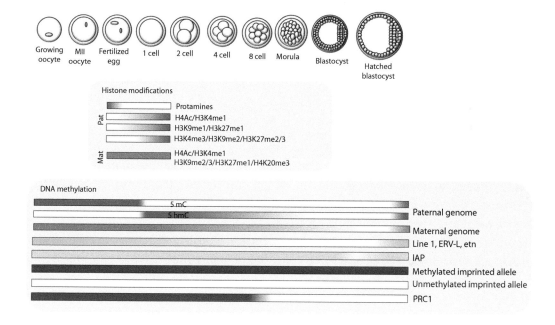

FIGURE 11.2 During preimplantation development, the embryo suffers extensive chromatin remodeling. Immediately after fertilization, protamines are actively removed from the paternal genome. The early pronuclear stages set the activation of histone modifications (H4Ac/H3K4me1), which are followed by acquisition of repressive histone modifications (H3K4me3/H3K9me2/HeK27me2/3). During the pronuclear stage in the maternal genome, both activating (H4Ac/H3K4me1) and repressive (H3K9me2/3/H3K27me1/H4K20me3) histone modifications are abundant. After fertilization, DNA methylation decreases to reach a low point in preimplantation morula or blastocysts (depending on the species). Paternal genome rapidly loses 5-methylcytosine (5mC) that is concomitant with an appearance of 5-hydroxymethylcytosine (5hmC, line in blue dotted) which is lost by replication-dependent dilution or DNA repair. Maternal genome undergoes a replication-dependent loss of methylation during the first cleavage stages. Many sequences like imprinting genes and some retrotransposone escape methylation erasure after fertilization. Line, ERV-L, and etn follow a similar demethylation process, while IAPs and imprinted loci are protected from demethylation events. DNA methylation and repressive histone modifications are removed during early cleavage development, and active histone modifications coincide with the initiation of embryonic transcription. All these epigenetic events make early development very susceptible to perturbation, like IVC, which can impact downstream development.

demethylation immediately after fertilization, while demethylation of the maternal genome happens in a sequential fashion; later, DNA methylation appears at the blastocyst stage (Figure 11.2). During this period, such epigenetic changes are very sensitive to environmental factors. DNA methylation is believed to be one of the mechanisms involved in regulating the gene expression profile of the embryo during its subsequent development. Suboptimal culture conditions during preimplantation embryo development could cause significant modifications of the DNA methylation in the resulting blastocysts (6–8) with unknown consequences. In this chapter we will review how IVC conditions are crucial to epigenetic regulation, including, but not only, genomic imprinting in murine, bovine, and human species, and how IVC impacts phenotypic outcomes in relation to genome-wide epigenetic regulation in early development.

11.2 *IN VITRO* CULTURE EFFECT ON MOUSE EMBRYOS

There are two main factors that can affect mouse preimplantation embryos and their epigenomes when cultured *in vitro* as revealed by generating changes in gene expression: Culture conditions and the composition of the culture media. Regarding the culture conditions, oxygen tension has been shown to be a main factor influencing embryo development and the resultant number of cell per embryo. There are two main oxygen concentrations usually used in laboratories around the world, atmospheric oxygen tension (20%) and physiological oxygen tension (5%). Significantly higher blastocyst production is achieved when culture is conducted under physiological oxygen tension than under atmospheric oxygen tension. This is because, the atmospheric oxygen tension is stressful for embryo development. However, this culture condition is still commonly used because of its reduced costs.

There are several studies describing how expressions of oxygen-regulated genes have important roles in the regulation of preimplantation embryonic metabolism (9). Mammalian embryos such as mouse embryos have the capacity to detect low oxygen tension and possess the plasticity to adapt to this environment by modifying the expression of oxygen-regulated genes (10). It has been analyzed whether oxygen regulates gene expression of glucose transporter-1 (GLUT-1), GLUT-3, and vascular endothelial growth factor (VEGF) in the preimplantation mouse blastocyst by culturing from the 1-cell to morula stage under 7% oxygen, followed by culture under 20, 7, or 2% oxygen to the blastocyst stage (10). Although development from morula to blastocyst was not altered, expression of GLUT-1, GLUT-3 and VEGF was increased by two- to fourfold in embryos cultured under 2% oxygen, when compared to embryos cultured under 20% or 7% oxygen, and when compared to embryos developed *in vivo*. To determine whether a high oxygen tension increases the frequency of epigenetic abnormalities in mouse embryos, De Waal et al. (11) measured DNA methylation and expression of several imprinted genes in embryonic and placental tissues from conceptus generated by *in vitro* fertilization (IVF) and exposed to 5% or 20% of oxygen tension during culture. This study showed no significant differences in development, but both oxygen concentrations resulted in a significant increase of epigenetic defects in placental tissues compared to naturally conceived controls (11). Moreover, Katz-Jaffe (12) analyzed the protein profile of mouse embryos produced under either 5% or 20% oxygen concentrations. Embryos generated under 5% O_2 more closely resembled *in vivo*-developed embryos, while embryos cultured under 20% O_2 conditions showed downregulation of 10 proteins/biomarkers. In the same way, Rinaudo (13) demonstrated marked perturbations in the global pattern of gene expression after culture under atmospheric oxygen tension as compared with physiological oxygen tension. Bloise et al. (14) analyzed gene expression changes present in blastocysts exposed to assorted culture conditions such as oxygen tension and demonstrated that atmospheric oxygen tension affected embryo transcription more severely, while physiologic oxygen tension have a lesser impact on blastocyst transcription when compare to *in vivo* (14).

Regarding the composition of the culture medium, a suboptimal culture medium such as Whitten's medium or presence of fetal calf serum (FCS) alters embryo transcription and results in offspring showing phenotypes with altered glucose metabolism and affecting their epigenome (15). These effects are equivalent to deficits in maternal diet affecting embryo and fetal development (16). For example, the presence of serum in standard culture medium affects embryo development and it is related to reduced pregnancy rate after transfer to recipients (3). Furthermore, it may produce long-term and transgenerational effects on post-natal development and behavior, including male infertility (3,17,18). All these failures have been related with altered patterns of mRNA expression (3). In addition, there are rising evidences that IVC influences the expression of developmentally important genes in the embryo (19) that are specially affected under suboptimal *in vitro* culture conditions as revealed when global expression patterns are studied through new technologies such as genetic and epigenetic microarrays (20, 21).

Mice are a good model to reveal phenotypic effects of epigenetic alterations by employing natural mutation like *Axin-fused* (*Axin^Fu*) or *Agouti viable yellow* (*A^vy*) model. These alleles carrying an upstream IAP element and the cryptic promoter in the LTR of the IAP causes aberrant expression of the *Axin* or *Agouti* locus dependent on its level of CpG methylation. A gradient of abnormal phenotype is caused by a similar gradient from an undermethylated LTR promoter (gene expression kinky tail and yellow, for *Axin^Fu* and *A^vy* respectively) to a fully methylated LTR (restricted expression, normal tail and pseudo agouti, for *Axin^Fu* and *A^vy*, respectively). In these mutations altered environment during embryo development affects epigenetic marks that lead to observable altered phenotype (4,22). Alterations in cytosine methylation or histone modifications during preimplantation mouse development are sufficient to provoke altered gene expression in adult animals and are reported to be transmitted to the following generation. Thus, preimplantation culture with fetal calf serum to provide suboptimal conditions altered the tail phenotype of *Axin1^{Fu}* mice, resulting in a significant increase in the tail kink phenotype observed in these mice (4). This was observed in association with reduced trimethylation at H3K9 and increased acetylation at the same residue, consistent with the phenotype observed after culture with trichostatin A. Culture alone, with or without fetal calf serum, also altered the dimethylation of H3K4 (4).

11.3 *IN VITRO* CULTURE EFFECT ON BOVINE EMBRYOS

Assisted reproductive technologies have been widely used also for breeding farm animals as a fast way to produce animals with the best genetic value. These procedures are especially useful in cattle, as selection for milk production over centuries has derived in a poor reproductive outcome. IVF permits that embryos from these selected cows develop normally in a foster recipient. Moreover, a great number of oocytes can be easily retrieved directly from the ovaries recovered at the slaughterhouses. After recovery, they are *in vitro* matured, *in vitro* fertilized and cultured until they reach the blastocyst stage (day 7), when embryos are usually transferred to a recipient. Embryo transfer following IVF show high pregnancy rates (around 60%) (23), as it is possible to select only high-quality embryos and transfer them to fertile and healthy recipients. However, the criteria followed to select the best quality embryos usually encompass only morphology observation, development timing, or cryotolerance, characteristics that might not consider genetic and epigenetic changes produced during embryo culture. Several transcriptomic analysis observed that suboptimal conditions of culture media affect the embryo during the most sensitive periods of development: Embryo genomic activation and early trophoblast differentiation (24).

Genetic and epigenetic changes produced during *in vitro* embryo development usually derive in disorders affecting subsequent developmental stages of the conceptus. Cytogenetic studies of embryos produced *in vitro* indicate that IVC increase the number of chromosomally abnormal embryos by almost two- to threefold compared with *in vivo* conditions (25). The most studied disorders associated with *in vitro* production of cattle embryos are referred to as large offspring syndrome (LOS) or abnormal offspring syndrome (AOS) (Figure 11.1). Characteristics related to AOS include incorrect placentation and implantation, an overgrown phenotype, congenital deformities, or even abortion. Several studies show that LOS arise from a perturbed epigenetic reprogramming during early stages of embryo development, leading to an abnormal expression of epigenetic regulation genes (26,27). The major wave of *de novo* methylation and the embryonic genome activation in cattle starts around 6–8-cell stage and it finishes before blastocyst stage (28). During this period, any subtle change in media composition meaning a suboptimal culture condition can affect DNA methylation leading to an incorrect embryo development or to impaired methylation patterns. For example, the DNA methyltransferase-1 (DNMT1) is more expressed in *in vitro* produced embryos than in their *in vivo* counterparts (29), so it is possible that methylation patterns in these embryos are affected.

Several approaches have been proposed to unravel the embryonic stages and the components of the media that could lead to an alteration of the DNA methylation profile. Different *in vitro* studies have indicated that bovine embryos are not subjected to strong methylation until 8-cell stage, but then the methylation level increases until they reach the blastocyst stage (28,30). This demonstrates that the embryo epigenome is affected differently depending on the developmental stages completed *in vitro*. There are some components that restrict the embryo development, as serum fatty acids, which affect the expression of genes related to metabolism in the early embryo (31). Supplementation of the culture media to improve the embryo cryotolerance has been widely studied, proving that it can enhance the embryo development (32,33).

Unfortunately, embryo development does not only depend on culture conditions. Various studies have suggested that even when the embryos develop within an advantageous environment, a considerable proportion of them will not achieve the blastocyst stage (34) or will elongate their trophectoderm at a different extent despite being in the same uterine horn (35). This is because the intrinsic quality of the embryo and the maternal-embryonic communication play a meaningful role on embryo development (36). Barrera et al. (37) investigated the effect of the oviductal fluid on the DNA methylation marks, showing that it affects to the expression of several epigenetic genes, as MTERF2.

Bovine embryos are usually cultured *in vitro* in large groups, as the interactions among them reduce the toxic factors in the medium. Nevertheless, in natural conditions embryos develop individually or in small groups, which makes the study of how individual embryos are influenced by the culture medium remarkably interesting. When culturing at low embryo density, it is essential to adequate the components (i.e., reducing oxygen concentration or excluding inorganic phosphate [38]) to improve blastocyst development. The addition of growth factors as transferrin, insulin, and selenium to the media has been proven to enhance individual bovine embryonic development, increasing the number of embryos which achieve the blastocyst stage (39,40).

Although there have been substantial improvements, culture conditions are yet to be improved for an adequate embryo development. This reflects the complexity of adjusting the components of the culture media to avoid genetic and epigenetic perturbations during early development.

11.4 *IN VITRO* CULTURE EFFECT ON HUMAN EMBRYOS

Assisted reproductive technologies are considered safe and effective so they are used extensively in human clinics for the treatment of infertility. Nevertheless, as mentioned above, previous studies in animals have suggested that some of the procedures employed (ovulation induction, oocyte *in vitro* maturation, embryo *in vitro* culture, etc.) can affect the genetic reprogramming that occurs during gametogenesis and early embryo development, leading to an increase in epigenetic perturbations (41,42). During gametogenesis, the genetic reprogramming of the primordial germ cells (PGCs) occurs before birth in males. However, in females, this process is completed in the late stages of the oocyte development which makes it more susceptible to alterations caused by the ART (43).

The mammalian preimplantation embryo responds to the variation of environmental conditions *in vivo* affecting the subsequent embryo and postnatal development. Some studies carried out in other species have shown that ART, including *in vitro* culture, influences the preimplantation embryonic development with long-term consequences (41,44). In humans, it is difficult to determine to what extent these techniques are the responsible of the possible epigenetic alterations. Many other factors such as the age of the patient, the fertility problems inherent to the couples that receive this treatment, and the diversity of protocols used in the different clinics, could also be involved (45,46). It is also difficult to employ healthy embryos, conceived naturally, as control of the different studies due to evident ethical implications. Moreover, the relatively young age of the children conceived artificially complicates the analysis of the long-term impact of *in vitro* cultures and ART (47).

Taking this into consideration, some studies have shown the effects of ART in humans. ART-conceived children have a higher risk of birth defects, increased rate of low birthweight, prematurity, and perinatal morbi-mortality than children conceived naturally (48,49). Ceelen et al. (2008) reported that ART children had higher systolic and diastolic blood pressure compared to children conceived naturally (50). Recently, it has been reported that DNA methylation differences observed between ART and *in vivo* conceptions are associated with some aspect of ART protocols and not simply by the underlying infertility (51). In the near future, it will be important to define if ART children present these effects in adulthood (47). Other studies have suggested an increase in the incidence of some imprinting disorders in ART children, that may cause Beckwith-Wiedemann, Angelman, and Silver-Russell syndromes (52) (Figure 11.1), but the absolute risk of conceiving a child with imprinting disorder after ART is still very low (53,54). Furthermore, it has also been shown alterations in DNA methylation and in the transcriptional level of a number of genes, such as those controlling growth (insulin-like growth factor [IGF]2/H19 and its receptor, IGF2R), in cord blood and placentae (55).

Many data suggest that *in vitro* culture of embryos may influence the phenotype of the offspring (56–59). The consequences of this potential shift in phenotype after IVC is to a large extent unknown, and it is unclear whether this have an effect on the long-term health of the ART offspring. The culture media used in ART is different compared to the fallopian tube environment (60) and there are a lot of parameters that must be controlled such as pH, temperature, O_2 percentage, and composition that interact with the embryo (46). Although most culture media share the basic components, the scarce information of the exact composition of the different commercial culture media make their comparison

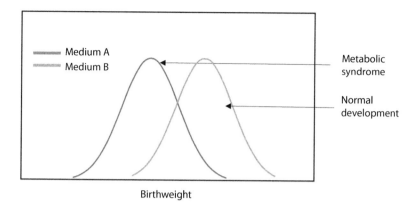

FIGURE 11.3 Effect of type and/or age of culture medium on birthweight of newborns. It has been reported that IVC of human embryos may affect birthweight and a correlation has been demonstrated between birthweight and adult metabolic syndrome.

difficult. Thus, it is still unclear how the composition of the media affects embryo quality and epigenetic, and gene expression in humans (41,46,61). Human IVF/ICSI oocytes are sometimes cultured and matured *in vitro* after ovarian stimulation of the patients. Immature oocytes are cultured in medium containing gonadotropins. Some studies have reported methylation of the H19 region (normally not methylated in oocytes) and demethylation of the region LIT1 (normally methylated in oocytes) in cultured human oocytes (62–64).

Regarding embryo culture, Kleijkers et al. (65) reported how the age of the culture medium inversely affects the birthweight of singletons born after IVF (66); and Ceelen et al. (50) showed that a prolonged embryo culture *in vitro* is associated with high odds of preterm birth (50). Dumoulin et al. (67) and Zandstra et al. (68) revealed that the type of culture media can affect human neonatal birthweight (68) (Figure 11.3). Other studies have reported variations in gene expression between the different media studied (65). The type of culture media is also related with a big placenta size (46), so it is likely that the culture medium affects embryonic development affecting the birthweight (65) and could alter growth patterns until two years of age (68). Ghosh et al. (2017) analyzed placental DNA methylation levels at repeated sequences to study the effect of ART and *in vitro* culture. They found that global methylation levels differed between placentas from natural conceptions compared to placentas conceived by IVF, and between placentas conceived by IVF in different culture conditions (different O_2 percentage) (42).

11.5 CONCLUSION

There is an evident lack of knowledge about the ART of embryo culture in humans and further research is needed. It is especially important in future studies to conduct experiments or collect data from a larger number of patients, using standardized protocols in order to confirm the effect of the *in vitro* culture on embryo performance and its long-term effects as well as the disturbances provoked at the epigenetic level. There is also a need for transparency by the manufacturers concerning the composition of the embryo culture media used as well as the scientific rationale behind this composition.

REFERENCES

1. Kohda T, Ishino F. Embryo manipulation via assisted reproductive technology and epigenetic asymmetry in mammalian early development. *Philos Trans R Soc Lond B Biol Sci.* 2013 Jan 05;368(1609):20120353.
2. Fernandez-Gonzalez R, Ramirez MA, Bilbao A et al. Suboptimal *in vitro* culture conditions: An epigenetic origin of long-term health effects. *Mol Reprod Dev.* 2007 Sep;74(9):1149–56.
3. Fernandez-Gonzalez R, Moreira P, Bilbao A et al. Long-term effect of *in vitro* culture of mouse embryos with serum on mRNA expression of imprinting genes, development, and behavior. *Proc Natl Acad Sci USA.* 2004 Apr 20;101(16):5880–5.
4. Fernandez-Gonzalez R, Ramirez MA, Pericuesta E et al. Histone modifications at the blastocyst Axin1(Fu) locus mark the heritability of *in vitro* culture-induced epigenetic alterations in mice. *Biol Reprod.* 2010 Nov;83(5):720–7.
5. Corcoran D, Fair T, Park S et al. Suppressed expression of genes involved in transcription and translation in *in vitro* compared with *in vivo* cultured bovine embryos. *Reproduction.* 2006 Apr;131(4):651–60.
6. Doherty AS, Mann MR, Tremblay KD et al. Differential effects of culture on imprinted H19 expression in the preimplantation mouse embryo. *Biol Reprod.* 2000 Jun;62(6):1526–35.
7. Mann MR, Lee SS, Doherty AS et al. Selective loss of imprinting in the placenta following preimplantation development in culture. *Development.* 2004 Aug;131(15):3727–35.
8. Market Velker BA, Denomme MM, Mann MR. Loss of genomic imprinting in mouse embryos with fast rates of preimplantation development in culture. *Biol Reprod.* 2012 May;86(5):143, 1–16.
9. Hammond J. The fertilization of rabbit ova in relation to ovulation. *J Exp Biol.* 1934;11:140–61.
10. Feil D, Lane M, Roberts CT et al. Effect of culturing mouse embryos under different oxygen concentrations on subsequent fetal and placental development. *J Physiol.* 2006 Apr 01;572(Pt 1):87–96.
11. de Waal E, Mak W, Calhoun S et al. *In vitro* culture increases the frequency of stochastic epigenetic errors at imprinted genes in placental tissues from mouse concepti produced through assisted reproductive technologies. *Biol Reprod.* 2014 Feb;90(2):22.
12. Katz-Jaffe MG, Linck DW, Schoolcraft WB, Gardner DK. A proteomic analysis of mammalian preimplantation embryonic development. *Reproduction.* 2005 Dec;130(6):899–905.
13. Rinaudo PF, Giritharan G, Talbi S et al. Effects of oxygen tension on gene expression in preimplantation mouse embryos. *Fertil Steril.* 2006 Oct;86(4 Suppl):1252–65, 65 e1–36.
14. Bloise E, Feuer SK, Rinaudo PF. Comparative intrauterine development and placental function of ART concepti: Implications for human reproductive medicine and animal breeding. *Hum Reprod Update.* 2014 Jun;20(6):822–39.
15. Feuer S, Rinaudo P. From embryos to adults: A DOHaD perspective on *in vitro* fertilization and other assisted reproductive technologies. *Healthcare (Basel).* 2016 Aug 09;4(3):51.

16. Fleming TP, Watkins AJ, Sun C et al. Do little embryos make big decisions? How maternal dietary protein restriction can permanently change an embryo's potential, affecting adult health. *Reprod Fertil Dev.* 2015 May;27(4):684–92.
17. Calle A, Miranda A, Fernandez-Gonzalez R et al. Male mice produced by *in vitro* culture have reduced fertility and transmit organomegaly and glucose intolerance to their male offspring. *Biol Reprod.* 2012 Aug;87(2):34.
18. Calle A, Fernandez-Gonzalez R, Ramos-Ibeas P et al. Long-term and transgenerational effects of *in vitro* culture on mouse embryos. *Theriogenology.* 2012 Mar 01;77(4):785–93.
19. Fernández-González R, de Dios Hourcade J, López-Vidriero I et al. Analysis of gene transcription alterations at the blastocyst stage related to the long-term consequences of *in vitro* culture in mice. *Reproduction.* 2009 Feb;137(2):271–83.
20. Giritharan G, Talbi S, Donjacour A et al. Effect of *in vitro* fertilization on gene expression and development of mouse preimplantation embryos. *Reproduction.* 2007 Jul;134(1):63–72.
21. Giritharan G, Delle Piane L, Donjacour A et al. *In vitro* culture of mouse embryos reduces differential gene expression between inner cell mass and trophectoderm. *Reprod Sci.* 2012 Mar;19(3):243–52.
22. Morgan HD, Jin XL, Li A et al. The culture of zygotes to the blastocyst stage changes the postnatal expression of an epigenetically labile allele, agouti viable yellow, in mice. *Biol Reprod.* 2008 Oct;79(4):618–23.
23. Mapletoft RJ, Bo GA. The evolution of improved and simplified superovulation protocols in cattle. *Reprod Fertil Dev.* 2011;24(1):278–83.
24. Sirard MA. The influence of *in vitro* fertilization and embryo culture on the embryo epigenetic constituents and the possible consequences in the bovine model. *J Dev Orig Health Dis.* 2017 Mar;4:06:1–7.
25. Raudsepp T, Chowdhary BP. Chromosome aberrations and fertility disorders in domestic animals. *Annu Rev Anim Biosci.* 2016;4:15–43.
26. Sinclair KD, Young LE, Wilmut I, McEvoy TG. In utero overgrowth in ruminants following embryo culture: Lessons from mice and a warning to men. *Hum Reprod.* 2000 Dec;15 (Suppl 5):68–86.
27. Young LE, Sinclair KD, Wilmut I. Large offspring syndrome in cattle and sheep. *Rev Reprod.* 1998 Sep;3(3):155–63.
28. Dobbs KB, Rodriguez M, Sudano MJ et al. Dynamics of DNA methylation during early development of the preimplantation bovine embryo. *PLoS One.* 2013;8(6):e66230.
29. Wrenzycki C, Herrmann D, Keskintepe L et al. Effects of culture system and protein supplementation on mRNA expression in pre-implantation bovine embryos. *Hum Reprod.* 2001 May;16(5):893–901.
30. Salilew-Wondim D, Fournier E, Hoelker M et al. Genome-wide DNA methylation patterns of bovine blastocysts developed *in vivo* from embryos completed different stages of development *in vitro*. *PLoS One.* 2015;10(11):e0140467.
31. Cagnone G, Sirard MA. The impact of exposure to serum lipids during *in vitro* culture on the transcriptome of bovine blastocysts. *Theriogenology.* 2014 Mar 15;81(5):712–22 e1–3.
32. Ghanem N, Ha AN, Fakruzzaman M et al. Differential expression of selected candidate genes in bovine embryos produced *in vitro* and cultured with chemicals modulating lipid metabolism. *Theriogenology.* 2014 Jul 15;82(2):238–50.

33. Leao BC, Rocha-Frigoni NA, Cabral EC et al. Improved embryonic cryosurvival observed after *in vitro* supplementation with conjugated linoleic acid is related to changes in the membrane lipid profile. *Theriogenology.* 2015 Jul 01;84(1):127–36.

34. Sartori R, Bastos MR, Wiltbank MC. Factors affecting fertilisation and early embryo quality in single- and superovulated dairy cattle. *Reprod Fertil Dev.* 2010;22(1):151–8.

35. Clemente M, de La Fuente J, Fair T et al. Progesterone and conceptus elongation in cattle: A direct effect on the embryo or an indirect effect via the endometrium? *Reproduction.* 2009 Sep;138(3):507–17.

36. Lonergan P, Fair T, Forde N, Rizos D. Embryo development in dairy cattle. *Theriogenology.* 2016 Jul 01;86(1):270–7.

37. Barrera AD, Garcia EV, Hamdi M et al. Embryo culture in presence of oviductal fluid induces DNA methylation changes in bovine blastocysts. *Reproduction.* 2017 Jul;154(1):1–12.

38. Nagao Y, Iijima R, Saeki K. Interaction between embryos and culture conditions during *in vitro* development of bovine early embryos. *Zygote.* 2008 May;16(2):127–33.

39. Wydooghe E, Heras S, Dewulf J et al. Replacing serum in culture medium with albumin and insulin, transferrin and selenium is the key to successful bovine embryo development in individual culture. *Reprod Fertil Dev.* 2014 Jun;26(5):717–24.

40. Augustin R, Pocar P, Wrenzycki C et al. Mitogenic and anti-apoptotic activity of insulin on bovine embryos produced *in vitro*. *Reproduction.* 2003 Jul;126(1):91–9.

41. Sunde A, Brison D, Dumoulin J et al. Time to take human embryo culture seriously. *Hum Reprod.* 2016 Oct;31(10):2174–82.

42. Ghosh J, Coutifaris C, Sapienza C, Mainigi M. Global DNA methylation levels are altered by modifiable clinical manipulations in assisted reproductive technologies. *Clin Epigenetics.* 2017;9:14.

43. Allegrucci C, Thurston A, Lucas E, Young L. Epigenetics and the germline. *Reproduction.* 2005 Feb;129(2):137–49.

44. Bouillon C, Léandri R, Desch L et al. Does embryo culture medium influence the health and development of children born after *in vitro* fertilization? *PLoS One.* 2016;11(3):e0150857.

45. Ross PJ, Canovas S. Mechanisms of epigenetic remodelling during preimplantation development. *Reprod Fertil Dev.* 2016;28(1-2):25–40.

46. Marianowski P, Dąbrowski FA, Zyguła A et al. Do we pay enough attention to culture conditions in context of perinatal outcome after *in vitro* fertilization? Up-to-date literature review. *Biomed Res Int.* 2016;2016:3285179.

47. Watkins AJ, Fleming TP. Blastocyst environment and its influence on offspring cardiovascular health: The heart of the matter. *J Anat.* 2009 Jul;215(1):52–9.

48. Wen J, Jiang J, Ding C et al. Birth defects in children conceived by *in vitro* fertilization and intracytoplasmic sperm injection: A meta-analysis. *Fertil Steril.* 2012 Jun;97(6):1331–7.e1–4.

49. Schieve LA, Meikle SF, Ferre C et al. Low and very low birth weight in infants conceived with use of assisted reproductive technology. *N Engl J Med.* 2002 Mar;346(10):731–7.

50. Ceelen M, van Weissenbruch MM, Vermeiden JP et al. Cardiometabolic differences in children born after *in vitro* fertilization: Follow-up study. *J Clin Endocrinol Metab.* 2008 May;93(5):1682–8.

51. Song S, Ghosh J, Mainigi M et al. DNA methylation differences between *in vitro*- and *in vivo*-conceived children are associated with ART procedures rather than infertility. *Clin Epigenetics.* 2015;7:41.

52. DeBaun MR, Niemitz EL, Feinberg AP. Association of *in vitro* fertilization with Beckwith-Wiedemann syndrome and epigenetic alterations of LIT1 and H19. *Am J Hum Genet.* 2003 Jan;72(1):156–60.

53. Bowdin S, Allen C, Kirby G et al. A survey of assisted reproductive technology births and imprinting disorders. *Hum Reprod.* 2007 Dec;22(12):3237–40.

54. Doornbos ME, Maas SM, McDonnell J et al. Infertility, assisted reproduction technologies and imprinting disturbances: A Dutch study. *Hum Reprod.* 2007 Sep;22(9):2476–80.

55. Turan N, Ghalwash MF, Katari S et al. DNA methylation differences at growth related genes correlate with birth weight: A molecular signature linked to developmental origins of adult disease? *BMC Med Genomics.* 2012 Apr 12;5:10.

56. Khosla S, Dean W, Brown D et al. Culture of preimplantation mouse embryos affects fetal development and the expression of imprinted genes. *Biology of reproduction.* 2001 Mar;64(3):918–26.

57. Gomes MV, Huber J, Ferriani RA et al. Abnormal methylation at the KvDMR1 imprinting control region in clinically normal children conceived by assisted reproductive technologies. *Mol Hum Reprod.* 2009 Aug;15(8):471–7.

58. Katari S, Turan N, Bibikova M et al. DNA methylation and gene expression differences in children conceived *in vitro* or *in vivo*. *Hum Mol Genet.* 2009 Oct 15;18(20):3769–78.

59. Nelissen EC, Dumoulin JC, Busato F et al. Altered gene expression in human placentas after IVF/ICSI. *Hum Reprod.* 2014 Dec;29(12):2821–31.

60. Li S, Winuthayanon W. Oviduct: Roles in fertilization and early embryo development. *J Endocrinol.* 2017 Jan;232(1):R1–R26.

61. Nelissen EC, Van Montfoort AP, Coonen E et al. Further evidence that culture media affect perinatal outcome: Findings after transfer of fresh and cryopreserved embryos. *Hum Reprod.* 2012 Jul;27(7):1966–76.

62. Khoueiry R, Khoureiry R, Ibala-Rhomdane S et al. Dynamic CpG methylation of the KCNQ1OT1 gene during maturation of human oocytes. *J Med Genet.* 2008 Sep;45(9):583–8.

63. Geuns E, De Rycke M, Van Steirteghem A, Liebaers I. Methylation imprints of the imprint control region of the SNRPN-gene in human gametes and preimplantation embryos. *Hum Mol Genet.* 2003 Nov;12(22):2873–9.

64. Borghol N, Lornage J, Blachère T et al. Epigenetic status of the H19 locus in human oocytes following *in vitro* maturation. *Genomics.* 2006 Mar;87(3):417–26.

65. Kleijkers SH, van Montfoort AP, Smits LJ et al. Age of G-1 PLUS v5 embryo culture medium is inversely associated with birthweight of the newborn. *Hum Reprod.* 2015 Jun;30(6):1352–7.

66. Kleijkers SH, Eijssen LM, Coonen E et al. Differences in gene expression profiles between human preimplantation embryos cultured in two different IVF culture media. *Hum Reprod.* 2015 Oct;30(10):2303–11.

67. Dumoulin JC, Land JA, Van Montfoort AP et al. Effect of *in vitro* culture of human embryos on birthweight of newborns. *Hum Reprod.* 2010 Mar;25(3):605–12.

68. Zandstra H, Van Montfoort AP, Dumoulin JC. Does the type of culture medium used influence birthweight of children born after IVF? *Hum Reprod.* 2015 Nov;30(11):2693.

CHAPTER 12

Epigenetics

Hope against Genetic Determinism

Josep Santaló

CONTENTS

12.1 THE SOCIAL PERCEPTION OF GENETICS

Our western society has a fascination with genetics thanks to scientific discoveries that took place during the mid-twentieth and early twenty-first centuries. Such attraction entails an increasing interest in the imaginary of our society, not only in new biotechnologies based on genetics, such as the newly developed gene editing techniques, but also in technologies with a strong relationship with genetics, such as assisted reproduction techniques (ARTs).

Interest in genetics and the transmission of our genes through reproduction has been a constant throughout human history, probably from the very beginning when humans discovered the relationship between sex and reproduction, something that, apparently, not even our closest relatives apes are able to establish (1). I believe this knowledge has prompted humanity to attribute an almost mystical capacity to reproduction as a creative force and has finally had theogonic consequences. In this sense, we know of the existence of prehistoric rites of fecundity embodied in paintings and sculptures where individuals appear with exaggerated genitalia, which were continued through the great historical civilizations full of theological and cosmological ideas in which reproduction plays a preponderant role (especially relevant are the Osiriac myths that relate reproduction to resurrection). Then, during the Renaissance and the Enlightenment, this interest was transferred from religion to science and, finally, during the second half of the twentieth century, the blooming of biology, and especially genetics, raised an unusual interest not only in reproduction but also in what, in essence, means: The transmission of genes.

Thus, the discovery of the DNA structure in 1954 by Watson and Crick (2) materialized and rationalized an idea from the studies of Gregor Mendel hitherto abstract. The idea of an "entity" that is transmitted from generation to generation, which shapes our physical existence, that even influences our personality and behavior and governs the evolutionary fate of our own species: The gene.

This rationalization of the idea is the scientific basis and justification of two concepts that would soon be derived spontaneously and almost inexorably from the initial idea.

The first one is the concept that appears in the book *The Selfish Gene* (3), the first edition of which appeared in 1976. This concept conceives genes as a force, written in themselves, that impels us inexorably to transmit them.

The second, in conjunction with the ideas of Social Darwinism, is genetic determinism. According to it, all our lives seem to be written in the genes, which act as the coryphaeus of great Greek tragedies, and which not only announce what we are predestined to do, but they impel us to it.

It is obvious that both concepts have been to a greater or lesser extent discredited and rebutted, especially in their most extreme manifestations, even from genetics itself. However, the attractiveness of its postulates and its apparent rationality have been maintained in the collective imagination and have a great influence in the perception that society has of new biotechnologies related to genetics.

The "selfish gene" concept has a major influence on how technologies, such as ARTs, are considered by society. It seems as if the idea of *the selfish gene* impels us to especially value "genetic parenting" and "genetic motherhood" as something fundamental, as a good in itself to pursue at all costs, even dismissing other concepts of parenting. This conception finally ends up by justifying ARTs themselves.

12.2 GENETIC DETERMINISM

The other concept, genetic determinism, is much more related to epigenetics and, therefore, will be the main focus of this chapter. In fact, as suggested in its title, epigenetics can be envisaged as the scientific justification that genetic determinism is completely false.

Genetic determinism is closely related to genetic essentialism. This idea states that genes are the placeholders of our own essence and are ultimately responsible for our own nature, aspect, even behavior and personality. This opinion is grounded on their perception by many humans as immutable, fundamental, homogenous, discrete, and natural (4) and it is often supported and encouraged by many news appearing in the media describing the discovery of new "genes for," that is, genes alleged to be responsible for human complex behaviors such as "gay genes" (5), "violent crime genes" (6), or genes influencing "the age you lose your virginity" (7). A remarkable example is the case of some variants of monoamine oxidase A that have been described as leading to more impulsive or aggressive behavior in humans, and finally appearing referred as "the criminal gene," "the warrior gene" or even the milder though bizarre "credit card gene" (8,9). This concept has not only been encouraged by irresponsible news produced by the media seeking to sell newspapers, but also by extremely serious initiatives such as the Human Genome Project (HGP) itself through statements such as "The information carried on the DNA, that genetic information passed down from our parents, is the most fundamental property of the body" (10). The coalition of science and media pointing out to the same idea has finally resulted in a decisive influence of the importance of genes and genetics on social perception, something pursued by the HGP to attain the huge amount of funding needed to carry out the project. This widespread opinion probably has had a final influence in the fact that, for many people, there is a closer association of the word "gene" with the concept of "fate" rather than with the idea of "choice," as stated in a work published by Gould and Heine (11). Although the authors cannot discern whether this is an innate association or it is the product of learning genetic concepts, this state of opinion surely would have had an important influence on this perception.

Such view, spreading and impregnating the opinion of our society, can have extremely crucial (even dangerous) consequences on our ethical perception of concepts as fundamental as human dignity, responsibility or justice.

12.3 THE CONSEQUENCES OF GENETIC DETERMINISM

Genetic determinism directly affects human dignity since it implies that, if true, "…our nature (or even our fate) is in the genes…" immediately leading to a debate which background "…[is] the dark feeling that biology is destiny, that what was thought to make up human dignity, mood, personality, freewill, self-determination, is determined by blind molecular and physiological mechanisms" (12). In summary, genetic determinism plainly denies autonomy, which is considered to be the groundwork for the Kantian concept of dignity based on reasoning, reflection, and freewill. Continuing this argument, the concept of responsibility gradually faints until almost disappearing, leading to a point in which justice is bearably applicable: No one is responsible for his/her acts but his/her genes. Unfortunately, this situation has already started and, in September 2009 in Italy, a man convicted of murder was granted with a reduction of sentence based on his genetic background making him more likely to commit violent acts (9). Moreover, this point of view has another side effect, which is that rehabilitation is not possible since true repentance is not possible (9). From this point, the argument is just one step far from justifying totalitarian eugenics practices. The only way to keep our society safe from these individuals reluctant to change is by avoiding their genes to reach the next generation (genes that are, ultimately, responsible for their misconduct). Thus, human beings are viewed as replaceable members of the species (or one of its sub-groups) so they have no longer dignity but a price worth to spare.

A second effect of genetic determinism on bioethics is that it opens the possibility of transhumanism, which has been defined as "a cultural movement that affirms the possibility and desirability of fundamentally transforming the human condition by developing and making widely available technologies to greatly enhance human intellectual, physical, and psychological capacities" (13). One of such technologies is the genetic modification of mankind to produce a "new human species" aligning with the postulates of "biological enhancement." It is obvious that such an aim is only possible if intellectual, physical, and psychological capacities are deeply grounded in genes. The ethical debate on Biological enhancement has recently acquired a renewed interest with the appearance of new gene editing technologies, such as CRISPR/Cas9. This debate should take into account whether genetic determinism is valid or not more intensely than what has currently been and whether changing human genes will finally have the desired effect proposed by transhumanism's leaders.

12.4 THE ROLE OF EPIGENETICS

Which is then the role of epigenetics in the bioethical debate? Epigenetics must serve as the scientific counterweight for such genetic deterministic ideas by acting as the scientific justification of the direct influence of the environment on genes and gene expression. A true scientific reality that explains how environmental factors can have an influence in our health, our appearance or our phenotype, exerted not by a sort of "mystical" influence but, at least partially, based on identifiable and measurable biochemical modifications. Therefore, epigenetics could be somehow envisaged as the materialization of existentialism. "Existentialism does not deny the validity of the basic categories of physics, biology, psychology, and other sciences. It claims only that human beings cannot be fully understood in terms of them" (14). In this sense, the aphorism of José Ortega y Gasset "I am myself and my circumstance" (15) implies that environment has a key role in human's personality whereas the phenomenon of human life possesses a double character: The "physiological" and the "psychological." Through epigenetics we now know that even the physiological component of our own identity has also two components: Our "inherited" genetic one and a second one, "acquired" or "semi-acquired," that is the epigenetic component. Epigenetics then becomes the first glimpse on an extremely complex reality where not everything is written in the genes and where epigenetics may have the "ultimate word." Therefore, human personality could be envisaged as a pyramid whose base is occupied by genes, the intermediate part is the space influenced by the epigenome and the tip is the realm of the autonomy. A human being is then the whole pyramid, not the base not the tip alone, and both parts are connected by the epigenome.

However, this scheme also implies some threats and dangers. The influence of the environment written on the genes and exerted through epigenetics could entail a new determinism which would be expressed a single step further. This "epigenetic determinism" could acquire higher relevance if epigenetic marks can be transmitted throughout several generations as recently suggested (16). If epigenetics influence can be transmitted to new generations and/or imprinted anew in our genes during early stages of pre- and post-natal development then a new scenario where deterministic influence in our lives would be composed of an inherited, namely genetic, determinism, and a partially inherited or acquired, namely epigenetic, determinism. This situation would bring the deterministic discourse back to the starting point by simply adding a new character in the drama, whereas the effect on the perception of autonomy and responsibility would remain wrongly intact. Moreover, it could have some implications in different aspects of bioethics such as, for instance, mother-child relationships. This is referred to the maternal responsiveness for proper development of the fetus (and young children, in this case concerning both parents) and its influence on the future life of the individual. An extreme example for this is the fetal alcohol syndrome, but other less dramatic situations can be envisaged.

In summary, epigenetics should help science to change the public perception of genetic determinism that currently seems to be deeply rooted in social beliefs, thus staying away from its disastrous consequences on the Ethics of advanced societies. However, epigenetics should also avoid the danger of ending up in a scenario where a new determinism is simply added to the old perception. It is not an easy task, but the essential trustfulness in science will surely help.

ACKNOWLEDGMENTS

The author wishes to thank Dr. Elena Ibañez and Ms. Lyan Santiago for their helpful reading of the manuscript. This work has received a partial financial support from *Red Temática de Excelencia sobre Bioética y Derechos Humanos: Impactos éticos, jurídicos y sociales de las novísimas tecnologías en investigación y reproducción* (#DER2016-81976-REDT) of the *Ministerio de Economía, Industria y Competitividad* of the Spanish government.

REFERENCES

1. Dunsworth H. What animals know about where babies come from. *Scientific American* 2016:314.
2. Crick FHC, Watson JD. The complementary structure of deoxyribonucleic acid. *Proceedings of the Royal Society A Mathematical, Physical and Engineering Sciences* 1954;223:80–96.
3. Dawkins R. *The Selfish Gene*. Oxford: Oxford University Press, 1989.

4. Dar-Nimrod I, Heine SJ. Genetic essentialism: On the deceptive determinism of DNA. *Psychological Bulletin* 2011;137:800–818. doi: 10.1037/a0021860

5. Rahman Q. *The Guardian*. 24th July 2015.

6. Hogenboom M. Science and environment. 18th October 2014.

7. Sample I. *The Guardian*. 16th April 2016.

8. Begley S. *Newsweek*. 13th March 2010.

9. Wilson D. Lack of free will due to genetic factors as a mitigating factor in sentencing. *Sentencing Conference 2010*. National Judicial College of Australia. The Australian National University, 2010.

10. Gilbert W. A vision of the grail. In: Kevles DJ and Hood L (eds.) *The Code of Codes: Scientific and Social Issues in the Human Genome Project*. Cambridge, MA: Harvard University Press, 1992. 83–97.

11. Gould WA, Heine SJ. Implicit essentialism: Genetic concepts are implicitly associated with fate concepts. *PLOS ONE* 2012;7:e38176. doi: 10.1371/journal.pone.0038176

12. Looren de Jong H. Genetic determinism. How not to interpret behavioral genetics. *Theory & Psychology* 2000;10:615–637.

13. Bostrom N. The Transhumanism FAQ. A general introduction. World Transhumanist Association. 2003. https://nickbostrom.com/views/transhumanist.pdf

14. Crowell S. Existentialism. In: Zalta EN (ed.) *The Stanford Encyclopedia of Philosophy*. Spring 2016 ed. https://plato.stanford.edu/archives/spr2016/entries/existentialism/

15. Ortega y Gasset J. *Meditaciones del Quijote*. Madrid: Residencia de Estudiantes, 1914.

16. Editorial of Nature Genetics. *Nature Genetics* 2017;49:815.

CHAPTER 13

Future Perspectives

Joan Blanco, Cristina Camprubí, and David Monk

I N RECENT YEARS, THERE has been a burst of studies analyzing the epigenome of gametes and its relationship with the transmission of epigenetic alterations in ART conceptions. Most of the studies have been done in spermatozoa because the simplicity of sample collection, the presence of high number of cells, which along with the relative homogeneity of the sperm epigenome ensures reliable results. Overall, studies in spermatozoa from infertile patients have suggested that sperm epigenome variations are associated with male infertility (Chapters 8 and 9). Unlike what happens in genetic causes of male infertility, in which an alteration used to be associated with a specific seminal alteration, epigenome variations have not been reported to associate with specific infertility phenotypes. Actually, similar epigenome variations have been observed from patients with infertile normozoospermia to severe oligoteratozoospermia. Moreover, epigenome alterations have been described for DNA methylation, transcriptome, post-translational histone modifications and chromatin protamination, probably because the mechanisms leading to the configuration of the sperm epigenome are interconnected.

Since many of these studies have been performed on relatively small number of individuals, without repeat testing or randomization, these disarranged results have been overlooked for routine incorporation into clinical practice as epigenetics biomarkers of male fertility. However, it must be noted that characterization of bulk samples only reflects the profile of a heterogeneous population of sperm and does not categorically echo the status of the gamete used in a fertilization event. In this respect, there is a need for the implementation of case control studies in well-defined group of patients, in a magnitude only obtainable through international collaboration. In the design of future studies, we should attempt to prevent false positive and negative results by conducting the studies using a large sample size populations with specific infertility phenotypes based on conventional seminal analysis. Moreover, taking into account the plasticity of the sperm epigenome, patients should be stratified by variables such as age, ethnicity, diet, lifestyle, and environmental exposure. The plasticity of the sperm epigenome has other consequences that must be explored in the future. For instance, we should consider whether we obtain the same results in different samples collected from the same patient, which would imply a fundamental problem within the spermatogonial stem cell niche and not due to transient environmental exposure. Lastly, as infertility is closely associated with genetic alterations, the influence of gene mutations that accumulate with paternal age, karyotype abnormalities, and single nucleotide polymorphisms associated to male infertility, cannot be ignored when looking for epigenome variations related to male infertility.

The study of sperm has also demonstrated that events occurring during spermatogenesis can result in an altered epigenome, which generates a footprint with a legacy important for early embryonic events (Chapters 8 and 9). Moreover, since the epigenome varies throughout spermatogenesis, a description of the progressive nature of the epigenome changes at different stages of the process would help to elucidate potential obstacles that may elucidate to novel etiologies of male infertility. While these types of descriptive studies have been performed in different species, their relationship to humans is likely limited, and therefore warrants investigation in man. However, this kind of analysis has several restrictions starting with obtaining samples, since testicular samples from fertile subjects are not easily obtainable and are ethically challenging. Furthermore, since several cell types are present in the human testis (somatic and germ cells at different stages of development) such studies would require an advance in cell-sorting methodologies to obtain pure fractions of cells.

The study of the human oocyte epigenome is challenging due to the intrinsic characteristics of oogenesis, namely: (i) Only a few number of cells are available for the analysis after the applications of exogenous hormones administration during the superovulation process, (ii) Cells are arrested at metaphase II and only complete meiosis after fecundation, and (iii) The epigenome is mostly acquired after puberty when primordial follicles progress to antral follicles. These limitations have restricted the number of studies described in literature and has therefore resulted in substantially less being known about the dynamic epigenetic process that occurs in oogenesis compared to the plethora of information we have for sperm. Accordingly, we have scarce data about how is the dynamics of the oocyte epigenome in natural cycles, or about the effects of advanced maternal age on epigenome variations that could be related to female infertility. Certainly, most of these limitations are very difficult to solve in humans and we will continue to rely on animal models for the imminent future.

For the reason described above, studies involving human oocytes have been mainly performed in medically ovulated oocytes arrested at metaphase II. Results have demonstrated a detrimental effect of superovulation over the methylation status of imprinted genes (Chapter 10). Nevertheless, there is a need for the improvement of methodologies to study the epigenome in low-input and single cell samples (which is inherent of oocyte epigenome studies); this is especially challenging for the application of high throughput approaches

(Chapter 5). Intriguingly, unlike sperm, single-cell technologies now make it possible to perform genetic and epigenetic characterization of the actual gamete used during ART cycles by assessing the DNA from the polar bodies of MII oocytes. Moreover, although studies have suggested an effect on the oocyte epigenome following the administration of exogenous hormones, there is a need to demonstrate if this detrimental effect goes beyond imprinting. These investigations could have important implications of the use of *in vitro* oocyte maturation, as well as the potential risks associated with oocyte cryopreservation that is routinely offered to preserve/delay the reproductive potential of women of reproductive age.

Epigenetic studies in surplus ART embryos are mostly directed toward the identification of methods for embryo selection. The epigenome of the ART embryo is the result of the convergence of the sperm and oocyte epigenome and the influence of factors related to the ART treatment. Apart from the detrimental effect of ovarian stimulation (Chapter 10), previous studies have demonstrated that *in vitro* embryo culture could be an additional cause of epigenetic variations (Chapter 11). Accordingly, it is extremely difficult to distinguish between the epigenetics alterations related to ART-treatments (ovarian stimulation and embryo culture) and those related to the patient infertility itself. Moreover, the study of the embryo epigenome has several technical and biological handicaps. First, as in the case of oocytes, the improvement of low input methods and single cell methodologies are mandatory to take into account epigenetic mosaicism within an embryo. Second, to clarify the influence of *in vitro* culture, there is a need of transparency by the manufacturers concerning the composition of the culture media used as well as the scientific rationale behind any supplementation. Third, since the epigenome of the preimplantation embryo is dynamic, undergoing genome-wide demethylation, it will be important to devise a strategy to analyze the embryo at critical stages of development, for instance in the two pronuclei stage, cleavage embryos and blastocysts. Fourth, how sperm/oocyte epigenome variations, and/or ART-derived variations accumulate in the embryo, or how gamete-derived epigenetic variants are reprogrammed (like the majority of the embryonic genome), still deserve more investigation. As with other medical disciplines, the consequences should only be uncovered through the implementation of randomized prospective case control studies in well-defined group of patients, something that is largely lacking in reproductive medicine.

Epidemiological studies have revealed a potential for multi-generation epigenetic inheritance in humans. These studies have been endorsed by recent data (Chapter 8) of loci that avoid reprograming in PGCs suggesting that transgenerational transmission of epigenetic-based diseases may extend beyond imprinting. However, the identification of demethylation resistant candidate loci for epigenetic inheritance is based on a single report; therefore, replication studies are required to identify common metastable epialleles in humans. Studies in monozygotic twins will help to elucidate those diseases with an environmental-epigenetic contribution and differentiate them from those with a genetic component.

Index

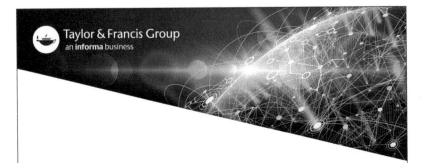